I0766909

Bridging the Gap Between
Between
GOD
and
MEDICINE

Joy Aifuwa, PharmD

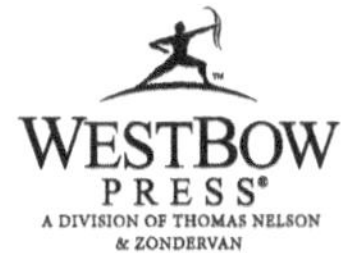

WestBow Press
A DIVISION OF THOMAS NELSON
& ZONDERVAN

This book is a work of non-fiction. Unless otherwise noted, the author and the publisher make no explicit guarantees as to the accuracy of the information contained in this book and in some cases, names of people and places have been altered to protect their privacy.

WestBow Press books may be ordered through booksellers or by contacting:

WestBow Press
A Division of Thomas Nelson & Zondervan
1663 Liberty Drive
Bloomington, IN 47403
www.westbowpress.com
1 (866) 928-1240

Because of the dynamic nature of the Internet, any web addresses or links contained in this book may have changed since publication and may no longer be valid. The views expressed in this work are solely those of the author and do not necessarily reflect the views of the publisher, and the publisher hereby disclaims any responsibility for them.

Any people depicted in stock imagery provided by Getty Images are models, and such images are being used for illustrative purposes only. Certain stock imagery © Getty Images.

ISBN: 978-1-9736-2748-7 (sc)
ISBN: 978-1-9736-2750-0 (hc)
ISBN: 978-1-9736-2749-4 (e)

Library of Congress Control Number: 2018905586

Print information available on the last page.

WestBow Press rev. date: 05/14/2018

"All things were created by Him, and for Him: and He is before all things, and by Him all things consist." (Col. 1:16b–17 KJV)

Contents

Introduction: My First Impression of Medicine

Before I begin writing on what inspired this book, let me first introduce myself. My name is Joy Aifuwa (my birth name of Oghogho is a Nigerian word for *joy*), and I was born on January 6, 1987, in Benin, Nigeria and moved to the United States at age eight. In Benin, as well as other developing countries of Africa, the availability of quality medicine was limited and sometimes scarce. My parents have shared with me that I was sick often as a child, but my memories of taking medications are few. One event, however, has forever marked me. I am not sure of the exact age I was when I was sick with malaria, but I remember the medications I took vividly. My parents gave me quinine, which came in a clear liquid form, and chloroquine, which was green. I remember gagging with disgust at how bitter the medications were. My mother made me take them every day until my treatment course was over. From that day forward, I vowed to myself that I would never take medicine again.

I grew up into my adolescent years with that same mindset and stayed clear of medications as much as I could. When it was time to attend college, I applied to schools with programs that would steer me in the direction of becoming a dentist. Since I was an athlete, I was offered a full scholarship at Felician College in New Jersey to run for the women's cross-country team and study biology. My loving father, however, was concerned about my having to apply to a graduate program after my undergraduate courses were over. Since he had been practicing as a pharmacist for over a decade, he recommended that I apply to schools with direct-entry pharmacy programs. I applied to the pharmacy program at the University of the Sciences in Philadelphia (now known as Usciences) and gained admission. I studied there and also ran for the women's cross-country team for four years.

My professional year of pharmacy school began during my third year at Usciences. I began to gain a greater understanding of how different medications affect the body, how the body uses them, and how it eliminates them. During lectures and labs, I learned about the factors that determine how effective a medication is, such as bioavailability, drug interactions, heat, and more. I was especially intrigued by how a naturally occurring chemical in the body such as gamma-aminobutyric acid (GABA) can be studied and chemically modified into gabapentin (trade name Neurontin) or pregabalin (Lyrica) to treat seizures and nerve pain.

I graduated from college in 2010 and have been a licensed pharmacist for over seven years. I have dispensed thousands of medications over the years and have witnessed first-hand what my teachers taught me in school: many of these medications are "maintenance meds," not cures, for most of the conditions they treat. Another thing I have observed during my practice as a health-care professional is that sicknesses and diseases are nondiscriminatory. They can affect anyone from the most educated scientist to the poor beggar on the street. I have dispensed medications to very bright doctors, lawyers, and people from high-profile families who are suffering from incurable diseases or illnesses. The stress and pressures of life today are leading factors for anxiety disorders, for which I have readily dispensed medications.

Even in my first few months of practicing pharmacy, I suffered from anxiety because of the stressful work environment I was in. I began to develop chest tightness on my left side when I worked, and I knew I had to do something different. Something had to change. I began reading Bible verses at work such as, "Fear not, for I am with you; be not dismayed, for I am your God. I will strengthen you, yes, I will help you, I will uphold you with My righteous right hand" (Isa. 41:10 NKJV) and "Have faith in God" (Mark 11:22 NKJV). As I did, the chest problem went away. I repeated this process over and over and have since applied it as well to pain in my joints, knees, stomach, ears, and head. Racing thoughts, depression, and fear have since been eliminated from my life because of this exercise.

After over seven years of applying this method, I have realized that medicine alone is not enough. People need much more help than what medicine can provide. Medicine by itself treats the symptoms but doesn't necessarily target the underlying cause and therefore is not effective alone. People need God in their daily lives to help treat their symptoms as well as the basic reasons for those symptoms. It's time to bridge the gap between God and medicine.

Chapter 1: The Origin of Premodern Medicine

Looking to Nature for Help

The innate desire for humankind to solve its various health problems did not originate in the twenty-first century. In just about every society, humans have looked to nature for answers to the medical problems that they encountered. Wherever there was civilization, someone always found a remedy—though not always a good one—to treat health symptoms. Although there are myriad medication therapies available today in the market, it was not always so. A few centuries ago, people had little to no knowledge of medicine as we know it today. Some sources corroborate that the earliest forms of medicine came from extracting ingredients from plant seeds, berries, roots, barks, or flowers.[1, 2]

Before the eighteenth century, ingredients from plants were incorporated into religious activities to promote healing. Since serious illnesses were believed to be due to spiritual issues, many groups of people used these ingredients along with incantations or spells to ward off evil spirits or to appease idols that they believed were responsible for their illnesses.[3] The

Japanese, Egyptians, Indians, Africans, and Native Americans all believed in the medicinal use of plants and therefore used them during their religious services. The Ebers Papyrus, a compilation of over seven hundred remedies to treat certain illnesses, originated in Egypt around 1500 BC.[4] The remedies contained mixtures of herbs that were used along with spells to cast out evil spirits and thereby relieve ailments.

Introduction of a Scientific Approach to Medical Issues

As the understanding of medicine progressed, people's concepts began to shift from believing that sicknesses and diseases were due to angry deities or evil spirits to believing that science could help explain many of the illnesses from which people suffered. In other words, they attributed disease states to natural occurrences and therefore began to study the human body. In ancient Greece, a man named Hippocrates, known as the father of medicine, introduced the concept of studying a disease by "direct examination of the living patient."[5] He pioneered a scientific approach to diseases, which is readily accepted in today's medical society. Many sources credit him as the originator of the Hippocratic oath, an oath that medical students must take before entering into the profession of medicine. Philosophers such as Aristotle and Plato provided more insight on disease states' being directly related to an anomaly in the body and not necessarily caused by spiritual entities. They helped develop the thinking process for solving medical problems; some of their key concepts are still used today.

During 800 BC, the Roman Empire emerged and had a significant impact on medical practices. Unlike the Greeks, who focused on finding solutions to diseases, the Romans were geared toward preventing diseases.[6] Roman physicians prevented illnesses by sterilizing surgical equipment before performing procedures on wounded soldiers. Some Romans, however, did adopt some of the Greek findings of the body. They also used "opium and scopolamine as painkillers, and acid vinegar (acetum) to clean up wounds."[7] As wounded soldiers were treated, knowledge about the body began to expand. Around AD 162, a Greek physician named Galen moved from Greece to Rome and became known as the father of human anatomy as a result of his extensive study of the human body.[8]

Resistance to Scientific Studies

Despite these primitive medical advances, scientific studies of the body were not celebrated or welcomed by everyone. During the Middle Ages, between the fifth and fifteenth centuries, the Roman Catholic Church was a major adversary of scientific research and development.[9] The church leaders considered many of the medical practices of the Greeks and Romans, which involved incantations, to be pagan; the Church therefore prohibited such practices among the people. Although they had the right concept of encouraging people to turn to God for healing through the practice of penance (repentance), they didn't achieve their intended results. In fact, some individuals were led to believe that their illnesses were a punishment from God, and therefore, many accepted their fates without question.

During this era, many of the citizens were illiterate, and because much of the literature was hidden in monasteries, people lived in darkness. Only the monks could read scientific articles, and by then "Greek and Roman medical records and literature disappeared."[10] Some scientific literature was retained in the Middle East and in certain Muslim cities. It wasn't until the Renaissance in the second half of the fifteenth century that things began to change. People began to die at rapid rates from infections caused by the flu, measles, and smallpox. One source reported that within the span of six years, twenty-five million people in Europe died, which was a third of its population at the time.[11] Another source reported that "within 20 years, the population of Hispaniola, a Caribbean island, dropped from 250,000 to less than 6,000 due to smallpox infections."[12] A term that is well known today, "the plague," or the Black Death was coined back then because of the massive number of people who died from the bacterial organism *Yersinia pestis*, which was transmitted by rat fleas.[13]

The First Vaccine

Widespread diseases created a demand for rapid solutions. In 1798, Edward Anthony Jenner published the findings of an experiment that he had conducted to develop a vaccine for smallpox.[14] He observed that milkmaids who tended cows that were infected with cowpox were themselves immune to smallpox, so he carried out an experiment to confirm his hypothesis. He injected a small amount of cowpox pus into little children and discovered that it protected them against contracting smallpox. Despite the resistance that he received from the Catholic Church and some of his colleagues, he became known as the father of immunology because of the vaccine's effectiveness.[15] His results paved the way for modern medicine and medical practices to emerge. As technology has advanced, so has the development of more sophisticated methods to create and administer medicine. However, the approach in developing today's modern medicine still resembles the approach of premodern medical practices in that active ingredients are derived by extracting or modifying naturally occurring chemicals, whether these chemicals are found in nature or in the human body.

Chapter 2: The Origin of Modern Medicine

A Greater Understanding of Bacterial Contamination

As technology advanced in the eighteenth, nineteenth, and twentieth centuries, groundbreaking discoveries accompanied it. After the microscope was developed, a scientist named Antonie Philips van Leeuwenhoek was one of the leading minds to begin examining microorganisms under a microscope.[1] By observing organisms that were not visible to the unaided eye, scientists were able to better identify the sources of some of the illnesses that many people suffered from; this then allowed them to develop enhanced preventive and treatment methods. For example, Louis Pasteur developed the method of pasteurization after observing that certain beverages such as wine, beer, and milk became sour after exposure to bacteria from the environment. During the process of pasteurization, the beverages were boiled to kill the bacteria and then cooled, resulting in an improved taste. As he continued his investigations of microorganisms, he and Robert Koch developed the germ theory of disease in

1870.[2] Between 1879 and 1882, Pasteur was credited to have developed vaccines for chicken cholera, anthrax, and rabies.

When Aspirin First Emerged

As the nineteenth century progressed, the number of scientific discoveries increased. Before the end of the century, the well-known and widely used drug aspirin was developed by Bayer AG, a German company.[3] The chemical formula of aspirin was inspired by extracting and analyzing salicin, which comes from a meadowsweet plant with the species name *Filipendula ulmaria*. Salicin is a form of salicylic acid, which is used to treat pain, fever, and inflammation, but it is harsh on the stomach.[4] This compound is also found in willow bark plants.[5] Aspirin, on the other hand, is a synthetic form of salicin and is gentler on the stomach than salicin. Aspirin formulations have since been modified further to become enteric-coated to protect the stomach lining.

The Accidental Discovery of Penicillin

Since bacterial infections were a constant dilemma, scientists continued to seek more effective treatment options. In 1928, a scientist named Alexander Fleming serendipitously discovered penicillin as an effective treatment of common bacterial infections, including *Staphylococcus aureus*.[6] He had isolated some colonies of *Staphylococcus aureus* in a culture and observed that they did not spread into the areas that had been accidentally contaminated with the fungus *Penicillium notatum*. Penicillin was further studied and later purified by Howard Florey and Ernst Boris Chain in the 1930s, and by 1941, an injectable form of penicillin was available to treat several types of bacterial organisms.[7] Today, penicillin is classified as an individual antibiotic as well as a group of antibiotics. Other medications in this penicillin family include penicillin VK, penicillin G, amoxicillin, ampicillin, and more. Today, this class of medications remains the drug of choice for many of the common bacterial infections.

The Use of Acetaminophen

As chemists manipulated chemicals to provide other pain-relieving alternatives to aspirin, a product named acetanilide was developed.[8] Like some of the man-made medications today, acetanilide proved to be very toxic to the body. Many people who used it developed a serious, life-threatening condition known as methemoglobinemia, a blood disorder in which red blood cells function abnormally and are unable to properly release oxygen to tissues.[9] If left untreated, this condition can be fatal. In 1948, a researcher named Julius Axelrod identified the offending agent to be acetanilide and suggested that its active metabolite, acetaminophen, be used instead to treat pain.[10] Acetaminophen was the actual pain-relieving, fever-reducing component of acetanilide.

Today, this finding has greatly impacted millions of people of all ages, as there are many formulations of acetaminophen for infants, children, and adults. All over the world, men and women can easily purchase acetaminophen, either as paracetamol, acetaminophen, or one of its brand names, Tylenol. In the United States, acetaminophen is widely distributed over the counter in grocery stores, drug stores, and more. It is also used in combination with prescription pain medications such as oxycodone, hydrocodone, and tramadol. In addition, the drug labels on many of the over-the-counter formulations of acetaminophen were recently modified to reduce the maximum recommended daily dose because of the risk of liver damage. Overall, acetaminophen is one of the top preferred agents today for fever, headache, and mild pain.

Discovering Antibiotics Produced by Bacteria

As time progressed, research for other innovative treatment options for infectious diseases continued to be a top priority. Antibiotic resistance increased, and other agents more effective than penicillin were investigated. The drive to discover medications that could treat more bacterial organisms that people were infected with led to a monumental finding, which was credited to Lloyd Conover in 1955. After studying two antibiotics (terramycin and chlortetracycline), which were isolated from bacterial organisms in the Streptomyces family, he chemically modified these agents to develop a widely used drug known as tetracycline.[11,12] What made his results unique was that he did something completely different compared to what was widely accepted in that era. Many other scientists understood that certain types of bacteria produced specific chemicals that prevented them from becoming harmed by other bacterial organisms. These chemicals were then isolated, purified, and, after adequate testing, used to treat human beings. Conover's discovery was unprecedented in that he came up with a method of replacing a chlorine ion with a hydrogen ion to synthetically create a more potent form of existing antibiotics.[13] Essentially, he was the "first scientist ever to make an antibiotic by chemically modifying a naturally-produced drug."[14] How profound was this discovery! People's lives were transformed for the better because tetracycline was effective against a broader spectrum of bacterial organisms that caused Lyme disease, hospital- or community-acquired pneumonia, acne, and more. Similar to penicillin, tetracycline is now both an individual antibiotic and a class of antibiotics known as tetracyclines (tetracycline, minocycline, doxycycline, and more). As impressive and groundbreaking as the creation of tetracycline was, the next several decades would reveal much more sophisticated scientific discoveries and inventions.

The Stress of the 1950s and 1960s Led to the Development of Modern Antianxiety Agents

Anxiety has always been a battle that millions of people all over the world strive to overcome. It was especially difficult for people during the 1950s to early 1960s. World War II had just ended, and Americans wanted to rebuild and advance their lives. The 1950s were known as the period of baby boomers; roughly "4 million babies were born each year" during this period, according to one source.[15] The drastic increase in population combined with a booming economy led people to believe that life was only going to get better, but they were sorely disappointed. As the Civil Rights Movement began to pick up speed in the mid-1950s, tension began to rise among the people. Stress was at an all-time high as the Cold War had a dramatic effect on the economy. According to one source, "Tens of thousands of Americans lost their jobs, as well as their family and friends, in the anti-communist 'Red Scare' of the 1950s."[16]

As the 1950s transitioned to the 1960s, more political tension was stirred. The threat of another war, the Vietnam War, loomed over the heads of political leaders, adding to the financial and social stress that the United States was already facing.[17] Anxiety escalated in the hearts of many Americans, which created a demand to research and develop effective medication therapies. Two antianxiety medications were already in existence—meprobamate (Miltown), a tranquilizer; and chlordiazepoxide (Librium), a benzodiazepine—but these agents were not favorable due to their side effects.[18] They were very sedating and were therefore not long-term solutions to anxiety. Also, meprobamate and some of the other tranquilizers had the potential for abuse and addiction, so their popularity eventually declined.

In 1963, Valium (generic name diazepam) was developed by Leo H. Sternbach as a more effective and safer alternative to Miltown and Librium in treating anxiety symptoms.[19] Valium works on GABA receptors to "enhance the affinity of GABA for its binding site."[20] In simple terms, it enables GABA to function more effectively as an inhibitory neurotransmitter. GABA is a natural chemical produced in the body to lower the activity of excitatory nerve signals, which play a key role in the development of anxiety or enhanced pain perception. The use of Valium or diazepam promoted less anxiety. Sternbach also developed another popular drug in the same class of benzodiazepines known as clonazepam, which is also effective in treating anxiety. These newer medications proved to be effective but still insufficient in lowering anxiety levels because they could not be used for long periods of time without causing some level of sedation, which was problematic in performing day-to-day activities. This concern paved the way for yet another innovative drug development: that of antidepressants to treat anxiety and depressive symptoms.

Melancholy and the Use of Antidepressants

The negative stigma of antidepressants has waned since they were first discovered in the 1970s to 1980s. Back then, people were ashamed to admit that they were prescribed such medications because to identify oneself as depressed had negative implications. As more people became affected by a state of depression, the need for effective antidepressants became pressing. A depressed mood had been previously treated with barbiturates and amphetamines, which were not very effective.[21,22] Barbiturates had sedative effects, while amphetamines were associated with insomnia, increased heart rate, and more. Imipramine, a tricyclic antidepressant (TCA), and iproniazid, a monoamine oxidase inhibitor (MAOI), were the mainstays in treating depression in the 1950s. These agents enhance norepinephrine and serotonin activities in the body; iproniazid prevents the degradation of these naturally occurring chemicals in the body, while imipramine inhibits their reuptake into brain cells, making more of these chemicals available for the body to use. Serotonin, otherwise known as 5-hydroxytryptamine, is one of several chemicals that affects mood.

As with some of the drugs discussed so far, the side effects of these agents became very problematic. Iproniazid was associated with kidney and liver toxicity as well as high blood pressure, while imipramine was associated with high blood pressure, constipation, urinary retention, and more. The need for an antidepressant that would mainly affect serotonin levels but have minimal effects on norepinephrine, which was associated with high blood pressure, led to the development of Prozac, with its chemical name of fluoxetine. Prozac, developed by drug manufacturer Eli Lilly and approved for use in 1986, became the first antidepressant that specifically targeted serotonin levels in the body.[23] It was primarily approved to treat major depressive disorder (MDD), and due to its antianxiety properties, it has since been used to treat obsessive compulsive disorder (OCD), bulimia nervosa, panic disorder, and more.

Additionally, other agents in this same class of selective serotonin reuptake inhibitors (SSRIs) have since sprung up. Added to this class are others with similar chemical formulas; the most popular of these are escitalopram, citalopram, and paroxetine. In your reading so far, you have probably noticed a recurring pattern, which is that many of the drugs that are available in the marketplace today are copies of chemicals that either originated from nature or already existed in the human body. Some of the medications used today to treat a wide range of medical conditions resemble the original chemical composition from which they were derived, while others have been so chemically modified that the body does not tolerate them very well. As a result, some of them have had serious, life-threatening effects in the body. This is not to minimize the tremendous benefit that these medications have had for millions of people all over the world. In fact, before the twentieth century was over, the groundbreaking discovery of one substance literally helped to save lives.

The Role of Cholesterol-Lowering Agents in Reducing Heart Attacks

As the incidence of new-onset heart attacks increased, researchers began to confirm a direct correlation between high cholesterol levels in the body and the development of heart attacks.[24] Furthermore, it was proposed that patients who were diagnosed with heart attacks not only had high total cholesterol, but they also had increased levels of low-density lipoproteins, or LDLs, a component of total cholesterol. Although fibrates and cholestyramine were already available to treat high triglycerides, another component of total cholesterol, they were ineffective in lowering LDL and consequently total cholesterol. Preliminary studies led to the discovery that a natural chemical found in the body, known as HMG-CoA reductase, was a major enzyme responsible for producing cholesterol components, especially LDL. It exerts its effect by first converting a substance called HMG-CoA into mevalonate. Mevalonate then undergoes several other chemical processes to form cholesterol.

In 1972, a group of investigators isolated a mold from a rice sample at a store in Kyoto, Japan.[25] Several substances were extracted from this mold, which was known as Penicillium citrinum, but one substance aroused great interest. This chemical was known as ML-236B, which was eventually called compactin, and it proved to be effective in lowering cholesterol in hens, dogs, monkeys, and humans. But muscle weakness and elevated liver enzymes were quickly linked with compactin. As researchers continued their investigations, a substance named mevinolin was isolated from another mold called Aspergillus terreus, whose chemical structure resembled that of compactin.[26] This product was termed *lovastatin,* and it became the first statin, a wide class of potent LDL and cholesterol-lowering medications, to be available in the marketplace for use to treat high LDL and total cholesterol.

Of the agents that are currently prescribed in this drug class, lovastatin most resembles its original chemical structure. Later, lovastatin was slightly modified to form pravastatin and simvastatin.[27] Some of the newer statins such as fluvastatin, atorvastatin, pitavastatin, and rosuvastatin are classified as "synthetic statins" due to further modifications of the original chemical structure.

In addition to these discoveries, many other medications were developed between the nineteenth century and today that are not mentioned here. These include vaccines for shingles, flu, pneumonia, tetanus, yellow fever, and more.

Furthermore, the availability of quality medicine has drastically increased over the past century as well. The options to choose from are so abundant that insurance companies have placed many of the medications that belong to the same class in different tiers or categories to manage their cost. In these categories, the least expensive medications are assigned to the lower tiers, while the more expensive ones are assigned to a higher tier. The purpose of these categories is to encourage prescribers to recommend the least expensive agents first or provide documentation to warrant the use of the more expensive ones.

In conclusion, many of the medications that are used today were first isolated from the natural environment, and after a series of tests in laboratories, other chemicals were derived from these isolates. Many of the drugs in the market today have their origin from plants and bacterial organisms. According to one source, "Almost one fourth of pharmaceutical drugs are derived from botanicals."[28] The same thing is true of many of the medications that modulate the release of certain hormones, neurotransmitters, and other chemicals in the body. These medications were designed to alter or enhance the function of naturally occurring chemicals in the body.

Who is the author of every living thing that exists? God is. Therefore, the practice of modern medicine is incomplete without the recognition and input of its original designer. God is still alive today, and His presence is clearly seen in all of creation, especially in the natural environment and in the human body. Furthermore, just as God has released solutions to various health problems through nature, He has released even more answers to common health problems; these answers are found in the Bible. Every word in the Bible is saturated with the healing power of God, such power that is not found even in the natural world. If you will read further with an open mind, I will expound to you the role that God plays in the healing of the human body.

Chapter 3: God, the Author of Every Living Thing

The Father, Son, and Holy Spirit Were Present in the Beginning

In the scientific world that exists today, if theoretical concepts cannot be explained through the five physical senses (sight, smell, hearing, touch, and taste), the concepts are rejected. In much of the educational system, students are trained to believe only what they can prove with substantial data. Biblical teachings are often rejected by the masses because people determine that many of the findings in the Bible cannot be supported. One area of teaching that will be addressed throughout this book is that God is the author of every living thing. This statement presents a problem to those with scientific minds because they can't see, smell, hear, touch, or taste God and therefore cannot prove His existence through typical scientific means.

How then does one prove the validity of the statement "God is the author of every living thing"? Most people may not be able to see God with their physical eyes, but the evidence of Him is all around them in creation. Romans 2:20 in the New

King James Version states, "For since the creation of the world, *His invisible attributes are clearly seen, being understood by the things that are made*, even His eternal power and Godhead …" (emphasis added). God existed before the creation of the world and, according to Genesis 1:1 (NKJV), He created the world. The verse states, "In the beginning God created the heavens and the earth."

Now before I go any further, allow me to first address this question: Who is God? Is God a force, a person, or a figment of the imagination? First, God is not a figment of the imagination. He has placed evidence of Himself in all of creation. All species of the animal and plant kingdoms reveal the diversity of God. Every colorful bird, butterfly, and flower reveals the beauty and creativity of God. The heavens, which consist of the sun, moon, stars, planets, and the constantly expanding universe, reveal the eternity of God. The gold, silver, diamond, rubies, pearls, and other precious stones on the earth reveal, on just a small scale, the massive wealth of God.

Out of all of God's creation, people are most precious to Him because people were made in His image and likeness and therefore reveal His godhead. When God created the first human being, Adam, He intended for Adam to resemble Him in spiritual and physical appearance and in character traits. Every human being who has since come into existence after Adam has been designed in like fashion. Genesis 1:26 (KJV) states, "And God said, Let us make man in our own image, after our likeness." God consists of the Father, the Son (Jesus Christ), and the Holy Spirit. This is what is referred to as the Godhead. This concept may be easier to grasp if humans are used as an example.

Humans are three-part beings made up of a spirit, soul (mind, will, and emotions), and a physical body. Likewise, the

Spirit of God, also known as the voice of God, is the Holy Spirit; the heart of God is the Father; and the physical representation of God is Jesus Christ. They are not three separate gods but one God made up of three components. The Bible says, "In the beginning *God created the heavens and the earth*. And the earth was without form and void; and darkness was upon the face of the deep. And the *Spirit of God* moved upon the face of the waters. And God said, Let there be light and there was light" (Gen. 1:1–3 KJV, emphasis added). Additionally, John 1:1 (KJV) states, "*In the beginning was the Word, and the Word was with God, and the Word was God. The same was in the beginning with God. All things were made by Him; and without Him was not anything made that was made … And the Word was made flesh, and dwelt among us, and we beheld His glory, the glory as of the only begotten of the Father*" (emphasis added).

When God created the heavens and the earth, the Spirit of God (the Holy Spirit), also known as the power of God, moved upon the earth with eager anticipation, listening for words to be released. (The Bible calls Jesus the Word of God.) When God said, "Let there be light," He released a part of Himself in those words, and the words took on a physical form. Suddenly, the light of God's actual presence, not daylight yet, came on the scene. As we read further down in Genesis 1, we see, "God said … and it was so" as He spoke the grass, herbs, fruit trees, sun, moon, stars, animals, and eventually humankind into existence. Although it's difficult for the human mind to grasp, God was able to create everything that we see because His words contain the creative power to manifest those creations.

By now, you may be saying, "Hold on just a minute. How can you prove that God used mere words to create all that exists on the earth and in heaven?" All right, I'll use humankind again as an example. Have you ever heard of the concept of a self-fulfilling prophecy? It's when you repeatedly say that something is going to occur and then it happens. During my college years, I had a friend who often spoke into existence the type of day that he would have. He would wake up in a grumpy mood and say, "I'm going to have a bad day today. Today is a bad day." He would start his day with that statement and, sure enough, his day turned sour very quickly.

How about another example? Many of you who have achieved great success in life use certain phrases in your daily speech such as, "It can be done," "There is always a way," and "Anything is possible." Based on these examples, you see that you can create your world with the words you use repeatedly. Do you know why you can do that? Because you were created in God's image and after His likeness. Your words may not be able to create a flower, but they can certainly affect your health and propel you into sickness or health, which I will discuss in further chapters. For now, let's dig deeper into what it means for humankind to be created in the image and likeness of God.

How Humankind Resembles God's Image and Likeness

To resemble someone's image means that you look like him or her. You share certain physical characteristics with that person. As I have already mentioned, humankind (males and females) are three-part beings. To be more thorough, humans are spirits made after God's own Spirit; they have souls (their minds, wills, and emotions) and live in physical bodies. Genesis 2:7 (NKJV) states, "And the Lord God formed man of the dust of the ground, and breathed into his nostrils the breath of life; and man became a living being." The spirit component of every human being was created in God's spiritual resemblance, and the physical body was formed from the dust of the earth. This explains why, when people die, their physical bodies decompose back into dust.

The Bible states in John 4:24 (NJKV) that "God is Spirit," but it's not the kind of spirit you're thinking of. He doesn't just float in the air like Casper the Friendly Ghost; He has a physical form. In Ezekiel 1:26–28 (NKJV), Ezekiel records the following: "And above the firmament over their heads was the likeness of a throne, in appearance like a sapphire stone; on the likeness of the throne was a likeness with the appearance of a man high above it.… This was the appearance of the likeness of the glory of the Lord." In other words, God is a spiritual being with a physical form that is identified as that of a man.

While the word *image* solely indicates a physical or, in this case, a spiritual resemblance, *likeness,* on the other hand, can be a physical or personality characteristic. When you have children, some of them may resemble your image or look like you. However, they may not always act like you (likeness). When God created Adam, He conferred upon him several of His personality traits, particularly the ability to dominate and multiply things.

Immediately after God decreed that humankind be created in His own image and likeness, He made this statement: "And let them have dominion over the fish of the sea and over the fowl of the air, and over the cattle, and over all the earth, and over every creeping thing that creepeth upon the earth" (Gen. 1:26 KJV). The inherent nature of humankind to dominate is evident throughout history. Where it has misinterpreted this mandate is in the object that it has dominated. Humankind (male and female) was authorized by God to have dominion over all His other creations, but through the course of history, human beings have dominated and oppressed one another, as seen during the periods of slavery. Others have taken the meaning of *dominion* to the other extreme and have used it as an excuse to mistreat animals. On the contrary, God intended for humanity to tame and take care of animals. He gave men and women the inherent ability to train them. Today, some people specialize in training domestic animals such as dogs, parrots, and even cats, while other people can train horses, tigers, lions, bears, snakes, dolphins, and more. Males, especially, have an innate drive to rule their environment and it is a God-given trait, although it has been abused by many.

The second-most important area in which humankind resembles God characteristically is in the ability to multiply things. Men and women can get together and multiply themselves in the form of children. Besides this obvious way, there are other, subtler ways that they multiply things. Men and women can multiply creative ideas, inventions, businesses, and more. They can think critically and creatively to take a little idea and turn it into a masterpiece. Artists especially have this gift. They can take a small concept and develop it into great artwork. When an inventor is determining how an invention should operate, he or she goes through a seemingly endless process of trial and error. Each time, he or she will try a different strategy or method to bring about a successful product. A businessman or -woman can start a business in his or her home and, within a short period of time, expand to a larger office and eventually establish multiple locations. Like God, humankind was never designed to think small or to stay small. Men and women were designed by Him to take whatever ability that they had and multiply it, expand it, and impact other people's lives in a positive way.

Everything on Earth and in the Heavens Belong to God

Living in a society where copyrights, patents, and trademarks are commonplace, people have often thought of themselves as self-made successes. Over the years, many have taken ideas, discoveries, or inventions and called them their own without giving credit to whom they originally belonged to—God. Some individuals travel to remote parts of the earth to obtain ingredients for food recipes to develop unique-tasting foods. Where certain foods are concerned, these secret ingredients are passed down from generation to generation in the form of a family recipe. Most of the spices that are used to flavor foods come from the combination of different types of leaves from various plants, all of which grow naturally on the earth.[1,2] These leaves are dried, processed, packaged, and later added to food to create delectable flavors that are commonly enjoyed by people of all ethnicities. Other spicy ingredients are peppers, which also come from plants.

While some individuals are connoisseurs of food, others prefer working with jewels. People have traveled to places in Africa where gold, diamonds, and other precious stones are prolific and have used them to create beautiful and expensive wedding, engagement, or anniversary rings.[3] One of my favorite things to do when I meet people is to look at their hands. Especially if I spot an engagement or wedding ring, I enjoy observing the pattern of the stones. Also, it is interesting to see how rings differ depending on the culture. I have a South African colleague who has a beautiful gold wedding band with a diamond in the middle of it, and as soon as I saw it, I fell in love with it. Nothing stirs a woman more quickly than when she is presented a diamond ring because it's such a stunning object. Do you know why these precious stones exist? Because God wanted to bring you enjoyment.

Last, let's not forget about machinery, especially vehicles. In just about every country in the world, they are available and readily accessible. What is unique about them is their diversity. I prefer driving small cars, while some of my friends prefer SUVs. During my recent trip to Nigeria, I saw what resembled yellow minibuses that transported people from one place to another. I had never seen these types of vehicles in the United States, and I was intrigued by them. Vehicles, regardless of the make or model, require certain basic products to operate: oil to lubricate engine parts, gas to get from one place to another, and metal, of which most of the inner parts of the vehicle (engine, rotators, brakes, wheels, and more) are made. Although this may be an oversimplification of things, the point is that the components of a vehicle come from products or raw materials that exist in nature.

Psalm 24:1 (NKJV) phrases it like this: "The earth *is* the LORD's, and all its fullness, the world and those who dwell therein." In simple terms, every plant, animal, human being, and natural resource was created by God and belongs to Him. Everything on planet Earth that you love and admire traces back to God. He placed certain characteristics in different plants so that you may obtain foods from some plants, while from others, you may obtain medicine. He designed animals in such a way that some can provide fur for fancy coats, scarves, and other clothing materials—even certain shoes. He uniquely created certain types of fish to be sources of lean protein for people who desire to be physically fit. For all of you who are bacon and pork lovers, He handmade pigs to provide food for you and bring you great pleasure.

You may have wondered why certain people don't look like or act like you; it's because they were not designed by God to be so. Some individuals are created extremely tall while others are very short. I stand at five feet and three-fourth of an inch tall, so I can relate. At a young age, I often read the *Sweet Valley High* series and so desperately wanted to be tall and slender like Jessica and Elizabeth Wakefield. I still remember reading those novels in middle school and hoped that I would magically grow long legs one day and become six feet tall, but that day never came. Just as people's physical features and personalities are different and unique, so are their God-given gifts and abilities. Some people can sing quite beautifully, while others sing so poorly that you secretly wish that they would never sing again. Other individuals have such mind-boggling athletic abilities that you sometimes wonder whether they are human. Regardless of what people look like or their natural abilities, the unique DNA of God is in them.

For centuries, people have fought over the ownership of natural resources. During the California Gold Rush, people traveled from all over the country and even from other parts of the world to dig for gold in hopes of becoming rich. According to one source, many of them "borrowed money, mortgaged their property, or spent their life savings to make the arduous journey to California."[4] Many of the people who risked everything that they had to travel to California never saw the fruits of their labor.

The presence of gold on the earth was first mentioned in Gen. 2:11 (KJV), where a land named Havilah is described with a river source (Pishon) originating from the garden of Eden. It mentions "…the whole land of Havilah, where *there is* gold; and the gold of that land is good." The second part of this verse discusses other precious stones: "There is bdellium and the onyx stone" (Gen. 2:12 KJV). Additionally, the book of Revelation paints a descriptive picture of a beautiful heaven—the place where the full presence of God and the throne of God resides. In Revelation 21:18–21 (KJV), the foundations of the wall of the heavenly Jerusalem are described as being made up of jasper, sapphire, chalcedony, emerald, sardonyx, sardius, chrysolite, beryl, topaz, chrysoprasus, jacinth, and amethyst. The city's twelve gates are made up of twelve exquisite pearls, and the "street of the city *was* pure gold, as it were transparent glass" (Rev. 21:21 KJV).

God deposited into the earth all the diamond, gold, silver, brass, pearls, rubies, and other precious stones that people have hunted for. In fact, He placed them there to be discovered. Psalm 115:16 (KJV) states, "The heaven, even the heavens, are the Lord's: but the earth hath He given to the children of men." God has given all the resources that are found in the earth to humankind to use and to develop goods, but they belong to Him. Besides precious stones, there are naturally occurring metals that are used to produce a variety of products today. Iron, copper, and lead are examples of such metals. Iron, especially, is a basic component in most machinery and appliances today. It is used to build cars, trains, train tracks, airplanes, buses, bicycles, buildings, and more. To further illustrate that everything in this visible world came from God, look at this book that you are reading. The pages in this book came from trees, as does any book or paper material that exists. The colors used to design your home originated from different types of metal pigments.[5]

Not only does every substance in the earth come from God and therefore belong to Him, but heaven or the heavens belong to Him as well. The heavens are classified into categories: first, the visible area that encompasses the clouds and sky; then the area where the moon, stars, and planets reside; and then the place where the throne of God is. A description of the content in the first category of the heavens can be found in Psalm 57:10 (NKJV), which states, "For Your mercy reaches unto the heavens, and Your truth unto the clouds." When you're outside and you look up, the clouds and the blue sky that you see are the beginning of the heavens. Although you may also see the sun during the day and the moon and stars at night, they are not actually in the earth's atmosphere. They are much farther away from the earth and make up a higher category of the heavens. Psalm 8:3–4 (NKJV) confirms that God also created this part of the heavens. It states, "When I consider Your heavens, the work of Your fingers, the moon and the stars, which you have ordained, what is man that you are mindful of him." Not only are the moon and the stars included here but also the other planets and all that make up outer space.

The next category of the heavens is not a place that can be identified with the natural eye or by a sophisticated telescope. On the contrary, it is an invisible place where God the Father, God the Son (Jesus Christ), God's angels, other forms of creation, and everyone who has died who believes that Jesus Christ is Lord reside. In Revelation 4:2 (NKJV), the apostle John gives this description: "Immediately I was in the Spirit; and behold, a throne set in heaven, and *One* sat on the throne." This person that John saw on the throne was God. God had taken John into a spiritual realm and allowed him to see the world of the highest heavens. He saw people and living creatures around the throne of God worshipping Him. He saw Jesus, who is identified in heaven as "Faithful and True" and "KING OF KINGS AND LORD OF LORDS" (Rev. 19:11, 16 NKJV).

Throughout the Bible, God gives many others access to this unique place so that they may write about it. Some of you reading this book may not believe that heaven is real or it may not appeal to you, but it should. It is a place that is more beautiful than you can ever comprehend. It is a place of laughter, joy, and peace like you have never known. Many of you have experienced such hardship in life that the thought of a place where there is no suffering or pain seems difficult to believe, but this is the reality of heaven. It is also a place where you will reunite with loved ones who have died who had a relationship with the Lord Jesus Christ. You see, God created heaven for you, not just for Him. It's a place where you will experience the tangible presence of God, see Him face to face, and hear His audible voice without any restriction. When you get a glimpse of Him, you will never be the same again.

In Isaiah 6:1 (NKJV), the prophet Isaiah says, "In the year that king Uzziah died, I saw the Lord sitting on a throne, high and lifted up, and the train of His robe filled the temple." The presence of God, also known as the glory of God, is so magnificent that it encompasses all of heaven. God allowed Isaiah to see into this spiritual realm by opening his spiritual eyes. This is one of the reasons people today have challenges with believing in the existence of God—because they can't see Him. For a person to encounter Him, that person must believe that He exists and have faith in what Jesus Christ did on the cross. God cannot be seen with the natural eyes but with the eyes of faith. If you're struggling to believe in Him, don't worry. Keep reading this book with an open heart, and faith in Him will develop.

Heaven is not a fictitious place but a real place where the presence of God is fully manifested. There, you will experience His love to the fullest. Revelation 22:4–5 (NKJV) states, "They shall see His face, and His name *shall be* on their foreheads. There shall be no night there: they need no lamp nor light of the sun, for the Lord God gives them light." Can you imagine what it would be like to have no night or darkness? We know what a little lightbulb does to a room full of darkness, but try to imagine being in a place with no lamp or natural light of the sun and moon. Instead, the light energy is coming out of God Himself! Think about how big and awesome He is to be able to generate all that light without breaking a sweat. This is the kind of person that I want to you to know.

Just as He lights up heaven, He can bring light to your life. If you will allow Him, He can get rid of the darkness that haunts you every day. You may feel like you're in a prison in your mind and may have felt this way for years. Bad thoughts may have crept into your mind often, and you have found no way of escape. Thoughts of suicide and depression may accompany you daily, but I have good news for you: they don't have to continue. If you will allow the light of God in Jesus Christ to enter your life, your life will change. As I am writing this, I see you out there, wandering in circles, trying this advice and that advice, yet nothing has worked. You know that you're missing something but can't put your finger on it to identify it. Wherever Jesus is, there will be clarity, revelation, knowledge, joy, peace, and rest. Heaven is a place that you don't want to miss. You can get a glimpse of it now as you develop a relationship with the Lord.

God is the reason that everything exists, including things that are visible and invisible. Because men and women are replicas of His intelligent nature, they are therefore able to discover, invent, and develop products or services. The advanced technologies from which most of society benefits should be first credited to Him because He made all the necessary tools and resources to bring about these advances. Although God's creativity, brilliance, glory, and majesty are displayed throughout the natural environment, He desires to reveal to humankind an aspect of His divine nature of which most people have little to no knowledge. He longs to reveal Himself to you as the healer and His Word as the true medicine. Before I go any further, however, I must lay a firmer foundation for why healing from God is necessary. Let's take a closer look at the natural forms of healing that exist today.

Chapter 4: Healers in the Natural World

Humanity's Innate Desire to Heal

Throughout the centuries, men and women have sought out various forms of healing to help those who were afflicted to get better. I mentioned in the first chapter of this book that groups of people would use plants, for medicinal purposes, in conjunction with their incantations to provide remedies for people who were sick. Regardless of how obscure some of these practices were, they highlight one very important thing: inside every human being is an innate desire bring healing to others. Although this book focuses on medicine as a source of natural healing, men and women facilitate healing every day through many other ways. Before I go any further, I would like to provide some examples of this with which most people are familiar. Healing can take many forms, but some of the areas where it is easily identified are in music and all other forms of entertainment, including the theater, movies, sports, and group gatherings.

Healing through Music

You may think it is a little silly that I would call music a form of healing, but you shouldn't be surprised. Right from the time of their origin, the melodies of music have had a way of soothing the soul (mind, will, and emotions) and bringing some level of calm to a person who has had a turbulent day. Although individual tastes in music may vary, ranging from punk rock to R&B, hip-hop, pop, classic, country, and more, each type of music speaks specific messages to the listener. As the musical artists write lyrics based on their own personal struggles and victories, this enables the listener to identify with the artist and, at times, provides hope to the listener. Speaking of music, I too am a passionate listener, although my artist selections have changed over the years. Music with an uplifting message can bring tremendous healing to people in ways that simple counseling may not because music has the power to penetrate to the very core of a person. It can transform a depressed person to become someone who will dream of better days ahead.

A practical example of this can be found in the Bible in 1 Samuel 16. King Saul had disobeyed God on more than one occasion and was eventually disqualified by Him from continuing as king of Israel. The Spirit of God departed from King Saul because of his disobedience, and he became very depressed. One of Saul's servants informed him that there was a young man named David who was skillful in playing a harp, so Saul sent for him. As David played, Saul became "refreshed and well, and the distressing spirit would depart from him" (1 Sam. 16:23 NKJV). Although its benefits may be short-lived, music can bring comfort to the listener and provide a temporary form of healing. This may be why some individuals spend hours at a time listening to it, to the point where they can quote every lyric in a song verbatim.

Healing through Laugher

There's a statement in the Bible that goes like this: "A merry heart does good like medicine" Prov. 17:22 NKJV). This statement couldn't be any more truthful. People need laughter, especially when feeling sick, because it too has healing effects. Laughing releases endorphins in the body, which makes a person feel better. The entertainment industry seems to comprehend this important fact as it floods us with shows, movies, or events to help us laugh more. The industry has been built by men and women who desire to bring people some level of joy in their lives, comic relief from their hard day at work, or just words of encouragement to others. Entertainment may be in the form of a comedy routine, movie, sports event, talk show, or reality show.

With today's vast forms of technology, finding entertainment is easy. At the click of a button, you have access to seemingly unlimited sources of entertainment. When I was younger, my dad loved watching *America's Funniest Home Videos*. As I watched the show with him, I laughed at the images that I saw, although I wondered why some of the contestants would risk their own lives just to win some money. To me, the risk wasn't worth it, especially as I saw people hit their heads painfully on objects. Even though some of the stunts that the contestants attempted were dangerous and others were a little silly, the show always had great ratings. In fact, the show is still aired to this day because the innate need of people to laugh remains.

If *America's Funniest Home Videos* never appealed to you, that's all right! How about another example that you may be able to better relate to, such as the *Madea* series by Tyler Perry. If *Madea* doesn't make a person laugh, I don't know what will. Although I am not endorsing the series, it's clear that there is a reason people spend time and money to watch or attend live comedic events. Comedy creates an environment for laughter; which allows individuals to take the focus off of their current situations, helps them destress even if it's only for a moment, and enables them to feel better. Although this form of healing doesn't provide a permanent fix, it is vital.

Healing through Poetry

What attracts people to write, express, and listen to poetry is that it facilitates a method through which people can release pent-up emotions in a constructive way. In a sense, poetry is a form of healing because it allows the poet to express his or her personal struggles or internal conflicts to an audience who can probably relate. When emotions are not dealt with over a period, they wreak havoc in the body, especially bitter emotions. As poets speak, they impart messages into the ears of listeners and provide an avenue through which their own emotions can be alleviated. They essentially help facilitate their own healing as well as that of others who have struggled with the same issues as they have. Poetry may exist in different forms, but the core of it remains the same—it serves as a method to express one's uniqueness in a way from which others can benefit.

The Innate Desire for Humanity to Bring Healing to Others Comes from God

Whether it's through music, making someone laugh, or poetry, people have an inborn desire to make others feel better, which is otherwise known as bringing healing to them. Although it is commonly understood that these avenues of entertainment play a vital role today, what is not commonly known or accepted is the source of this innate desire. Secular humanism would have you believe that men and women are good by themselves and can exist without God, but this isn't true. Before humankind began to develop ways to help one another deal with their physical or emotional illnesses, they looked to the things that God created for answers. As mentioned in earlier chapters, people from different ethnic backgrounds began to discover the medicinal purposes of plants at an early period. The more they studied the natural environment, which God created, the more of His treasure field was uncovered. As brilliant as researchers are today, they have not been able to identify all of God's unlimited resources that are found in the earth, nor have they made full use of the ones that have already been identified. The desire to take the resources found in the natural environment, reproduce or modify them, and then sell them as different products to improve the lives of others came straight from the heart of God.

God created you in His image and likeness, and just as Jesus Christ went about healing people who were sick, He's placed that same desire in you. This is the reason there are facilities where people with problems such as drug or alcohol addiction can go, spend a few days or an extended period, and get healed in the area that they are struggling to overcome. In an environment like this, people experiencing addiction can receive counseling, become part of a support group, and talk through the process of their addiction to change their mind-sets and habits. When they then leave that facility, they have a different outlook; and if they are consistent, they will become completely free of the desire to regress to former habits. This is one example of how people today apply the nature of God in them to bring healing to others, without realizing it.

As I continue discussing the different types of healing that exist in the natural world, I certainly cannot leave out hospitals. Although there are a lot of politics involved today, hospitals were originally designed as places where people who were sick could been seen by a health-care professional, primarily a doctor, and receive treatment. Some of the people who walk into a hospital today may not have urgent problems, while others are in a life-or-death situation. Hospitals are supposed to provide a safe, well-controlled environment where people who are ill can be evaluated, diagnosed, and prescribed medications or treatments to facilitate healing in their bodies. It is also a place where qualified individuals can receive major or minor surgery, and afterwards, they are provided rooms in which to sleep and recover until they are well enough to go home.

As you can see, the passion to bring healing to others is prevalent today, and this passion can only come from God. Imagine the sleepless nights and the years of training that doctors must go through before they are fully equipped to practice. Although this profession is highly rewarding financially and socially, these factors are not what drive true doctors, or other health-care professionals for that matter, to endure the process of training. Many of them persevere through the arduous journey of preparation because they genuinely desire to help people get better. They are passionate about what they do, even at the cost of their own marriages and families at times.

Healing Is Not Strange to Society

As you have read so far, the word *healing* is not strange to the natural world and should not seem strange to you. It is incorporated in every society across the globe, although it may exist in different forms. Can you think of other signs of healing that exist in the natural world where you live? Without having to look too far, you can easily spot them as you walk down the street. You may wonder what I mean. I am referring to the names of businesses and some of the services that they offer.

Some businesses may attach the word *wellness* to their business names or services to indicate to potential customers that what they have to offer will help those customers become healthier or well. The word *wellness* is synonymous with *healing* because, as a person is restored from an unwell (unhealthy) state to a well (healthy) state, healing has taken place in that person's body. Remember that the definition of *healing*, according to *Merriam-Webster's Dictionary*, is "to make sound or whole; to make well again."[1] Wellness or healing is prevalent as you look at some of the services and goods offered by drug stores, grocery stores, spas or other places to get massages, and more. At a company where I once worked, the "wellness package" that we offered included health screenings, a free consultation with a health-care professional, genetic diagnostic tests, immunizations, and more.

Beware of Slipping into Extremes

In other places, healing is marketed in the form of meditation, mind detox, and more. I am not referring to meditating on the Word of God or using biblical principles to change your thinking from a negative to a positive way. I am addressing practices where certain spiritual beliefs that are not of God are applied to a person's thinking to convert his or her way of thinking. You have even heard of someone describing another person as having "positive energy" or "negative energy" and the need to get rid of that negative energy. Without going into any further detail, I would like to caution you to be aware that there are many phony substitutes of the real healing that comes from God and from the things that He created. There are some individuals who have twisted certain aspects of healing and converted them into something that is dangerous to participate in. If you stick with what the Bible says about how to obtain healing, which is primarily through the Word of God and from the foods and plants that He created, you will be safe.

A Look at the Current Health-Care System

As the need to provide quality services to patients increased, this placed a demand for more highly skilled professionals to be included in the health-care team. Although insurance companies also play a role here, I am going to focus on the individuals who have direct contact with patients. When you visit a hospital, especially if it is a teaching hospital, you will see various uniforms identifying different groups of people who make up a health-care team. Some may wear scrubs with a name tag of a distinct color to identify themselves as doctors or nurses, while others may wear a white coat with a name tag to identify themselves as doctors, pharmacists, or other professionals. The point that I am trying to make here is that doctors, nurses, physician's assistants, pharmacists, dieticians, social workers, psychiatrists, and other health-care professionals and workers all play a vital role in bringing healing to sick individuals who are under their care. How? This is achieved by the types of services that each one of them offers, which are based on their individual level of expertise. As all of them work together, they cover a wide scope of areas that need to be addressed to help a person become whole.

Health-Care Professionals Are Ministers of Healing

During one of his daily broadcasts, I heard one of my spiritual fathers, Kenneth Copeland, call his personal physician a "minister of healing," and that statement struck a chord with me. If a doctor is a minister of healing because his or her occupation involves helping sick people to get well, then this term can also be applied to any health-care professional who plays a role in patients' recovery processes. When you see the word *minister* in this context, I'm not referring to the person to whom you listen preach or teach on Sundays. In its simplest definition, to *minister* to someone is to give some of what you have to that person. This gift may be in the form of tangible objects such as money and goods or something intangible like knowledge of a thing. One definition that spells it out perfectly comes from the *Merriam-Webster Dictionary*, where it defines the verb *minister* as "to give aid or service."[2] How are doctors, doctor assistants, nurses, pharmacists, and other health-care workers ministers of healing? Good question. Let's look at some of their roles.

When a patient is sick and attends a hospital or a health clinic, he or she is asked a series of questions by a nurse or a physician to help identify the real reason he or she isn't feeling well. The hospital personnel may run a few diagnostic tests to rule out certain illnesses, and depending on the level of severity, the person may either be hospitalized or sent home within a few hours. In the case of hospitalized patients, they are assigned a room and a personal nurse who will look after them. As they wait to be further evaluated by a physician, an assigned nurse cares for them, making sure that the proper amounts of blood have been drawn and sent to the lab. Nurses also see to it that their patients are as comfortable as possible; are receiving the necessary fluids, food, and medications; and are able to use the bathroom, with assistance if needed. They also help clean a patient's wounds daily, rotate him or her daily to prevent bedsores, and maintain an adequate room environment to prevent opportunistic infections. In a nutshell, nurses care for the minute needs of patients during their hospital stays and, in this sense, aid the patient's healing process.

As nurses continue to carry out their daily tasks, the assigned physicians read the notes that are documented in their patients' charts and visit each patient's room. At least once a day, a doctor will make rounds, a medical term that simply means to visit many or all of the hospitalized patients assigned to him or her. During these rounds, there may be a team consisting of an attending physician (a more experienced doctor), a resident (a doctor still in training), pharmacists, and pharmacy students/residents. Physicians may ask some questions and then perform physical evaluations of each of their patients. They may listen to a person's heart and lungs or may simply examine the area of concern. After observation, they write a few comments inside each patient's chart to make the necessary adjustments in his or her medical care.

Doctors specialize in the diagnosis of a disease state and will use their expertise to determine what's wrong with the patient and prescribe medications to alleviate the symptoms of the illness or disease, if needed. Furthermore, doctors may use literary references to help ensure that they are making the most accurate recommendation because the wrong prescribed medicine may impair a patient's health, while the right one may help to speed up a patient's recovery process. He or she may prescribe a different antibiotic, lengthen or shorten a person's stay, or place a request for a consultation from a different health-care provider. The regimens that hospitalized patients must adhere to may determine how quickly their bodies return to normal health.

I've illustrated the role of nurses and doctors in facilitating a person's healing, but how about pharmacists? Some of you have formed an opinion of pharmacists as "glorified technicians," and in a sense, this is true because their initial responsibilities as pharmacy students are those of a technician. What you may not know about them is their important role in a person's healing process. Since I have much more experience in a retail or community setting than in a hospital setting, I will provide you a description of a good pharmacist. (I say *good* because there are some nasty ones who have no business being around people, period.)

Having worked in a retail setting for almost ten years (two years as a student and almost eight years as a pharmacist), I can say from personal experience that pharmacists are ministers of healing. They have direct access to people and are not necessarily restricted in the amount of time that they can spend with them (unless they get backed up with their work). Each prescribed medication that is dispensed by the pharmacist must be accompanied with corresponding paperwork. The paperwork usually contains the name, strength, and direction of a medication, as well as its common side effects. As pharmacists review the medication profile of the patient (although the information can be limited), they can identify potential drug-interactions or duplication of therapy, both of which may bring harm to the patient. As patients pick up their medications, they are usually asked if they would like to consult with a pharmacist. This is another area in which pharmacists can have tremendous influence in a person's well-being. As they provide counsel where appropriate, they can intercept potentially dangerous events from occurring, such as a customer who is prescribed a sleep medication and then picks up an over-the-counter sleep remedy as well. Sometimes a customer may come in and want to unload all of his or her day's stress on someone, and the pharmacist is there to listen, take the heat, or provide sound counsel without responding unprofessionally.

An Unforgettable Story

On a lighter note, I have countless stories that I could share about my encounters with some of my customers, but one stands out distinctly in my mind, and I probably will never forget it. On this day, I was filling in at a store different from my usual location. A customer's relative came to pick up a medication that I had filled that day. I was not forewarned that the customer had made a special request for a specific drug manufacturer, so I dispensed the one that the pharmacy had in stock. This occurred on a Saturday, and what I thought would be an easy nine-hour shift quickly turned out to be a day of horror. When the customer's relative got home and delivered the medicine, the customer became furious and called me at the store. I apologized (every pharmacist must be proficient in apologizing even for mistakes that are not their own) to her and quickly realized that her regular pharmacist had not ordered the medicine from the manufacturer that she had requested.

She became so angry with me that she called me a derogatory and racially charged word and hung the phone up on me several times as I attempted to rectify the situation. During my last attempt to reach her, she threatened to call the police on me if I called her back. I laugh now as I recall this event, but it wasn't funny when it happened. I remember how red my ears and palms became as I processed what had just occurred. I eventually calmed myself down, forgave her in my heart, and went about my business for the rest of my shift. Fortunately for me, the story ended well.

About thirty minutes before closing, she called me back and—I must admit—I really didn't want to speak to her. She begged me for forgiveness and shared that she was suffering from some level of depression. I have had to forgive rude customers before, but she said something that struck me: "You are such a nice person. I am so sorry for what I said. There was such an urge in me to call you back and apologize." The point I am trying to make is that at that moment, I had the choice to refuse her apology, which may have worsened her depressed feelings, or say an encouraging word to bring her comfort and some level of healing to her current emotions. I chose the latter option.

Pharmacists can steer a customer in the right direction or the wrong direction based on the recommendations or advice that they provide. Good advice can lead to improved lifestyle habits and health, while bad advice may sink a customer further down a hole. During many encounters with patients, which may be daily to monthly, a pharmacist dispenses medications to them, answers their questions, and may speak comforting words to their troubled lives. All of this put together helps facilitate the emotional and physical healing of a customer.

Although I am not going into detail about these additional groups, there are other health-care professionals and workers who play vital roles in bringing a person from an unwell state to a well state. These include social workers, counselors, psychiatrists, and all other health-care providers. In a sense, they too are ministers of healing because their primary role is assisting a patient's recovery process.

The Disconnect

Despite their great potential, many health-care workers today fall short of fulfilling their true assignment to aid in the healing of their patients for various reasons. The first major reason is that they have shut God out of their personal lives and professional practices. Many of them have no personal relationship with the Lord Jesus Christ and therefore go about their daily activities based on intellect alone. One thing that never ceases to amaze me is the fact that many institutions cleave firmly to journal articles, clinical trials, textbooks, and all other forms of medical literature as true sources of information and reject everything outside of that. If it cannot be explained with scientific studies, many health professionals conclude that it has no grounds for acceptance. However, these are the same people who will admit that they don't have all the answers to the health problems that are faced today. In the medical world, you will hear the term *evidence-based medicine* thrown around a lot and even touted proudly.

What is evidence-based medicine, anyway? It simply refers to medical findings that can be corroborated with appropriate and adequate scientific research. For example, if a group of individuals claim that the medicine they have developed is effective in lowering cholesterol, then they must take a series of steps to prove the veracity of their claim. This involves performing experiments to test their hypothesis, developing clinical trials to identify the demographics this medication is effective in treating, writing an article about their findings that addresses the positive and negative results of their experiments, and eventually submitting this data for evaluation. Although I have given an abbreviated version of the process, the principle stands true.

Evidence-based medicine is necessary, and without it, more unnecessary deaths might occur. Drug manufacturers should provide substantial data to authenticate their claims. This requirement by the US Food and Drug Administration (FDA) has also greatly reduced the likelihood of greedy drug manufacturers who just want to make money developing substandard medications (I say "greatly reduced" but not "altogether eliminated" this problem). If evidence-based medicine is great and vital, then what's the problem? The problem is that men and women have grown to rely on "evidence" from medical articles but rejected God, the One who created all that they see, hear, taste, touch, and smell.

When I was in pharmacy school, a few of my professors would refer to our pharmacotherapy text book as our "bible," implying that we were to pay close attention to what we read in it the same way one would pay close attention to the Holy Bible. I remember thinking how completely contradictory this statement was. They didn't mind that we memorized and quoted literature as long as it was the literature that they had approved. I don't blame these professors, however, because this is how they were trained by their instructors.

By shutting God completely out of their professional practices, health-care workers have unknowingly limited their effectiveness. Many of them mean well and have a heart to help their patients, but how can they fully accomplish their role with a deformity? It's like trying to wash dishes manually but your arms have been cut off. You may have a passion to soak your dishes in hot water and wipe them until they sparkle, but if you don't have arms, you are simply limited as to what you'll be able to do. You may think that this illustration is a little silly and maybe it is, but do you see the point that is being made? You cannot attempt to bring healing to a dying world by relying on books or personal experiences alone. You discover how to help others get better by consulting the One who created the natural environment and the human body, from which came the inspiration to develop modern medicine!

Hearing from God for Your Patient

Allow me to give you another practical example of what I am saying. Let's say that you're a doctor and a patient steps into your office or clinic with terrible pain. What's the first thing that you may do? You or your nurse may ask the person a series of questions to identify or rule out certain possibilities and may perform a physical exam of your own. Eventually, after running some tests, considering the patient's chief complaint, and calling on your medical expertise, you make a recommendation. Your approach towards this person's pain is by the book and correct. However, suppose the patient follows your instructions and gets worse. What do you do next?

You may refer to your medical literature and, based on it, change your diagnosis and prescribe something else. Again, what you've done is right. Here's where I will introduce something that you may not have learned in your medical training. Many health problems stem from issues that are beneath the surface and are not easily identifiable without a relationship with Jesus Christ. As you're listening to the patient complain about pain in an area, the Holy Spirit may speak to your heart that the patient is not telling you something—a vital piece of information that has been left out. He may tell you to ask the patient a different type of question so that you can quickly identify the root cause, instead of relying on trial and error. Instead of recommending one drug, He may lead you to prescribe a different one, and much to your surprise, it will quicken the person's recovery process.

You may read this and ask, "How can I do what you are suggesting when my schedule is so tight?" Start small. Begin by spending the first fifteen to thirty minutes of your day in prayer and fellowship with God. Read a chapter of the Bible daily, and ask Him to reveal Himself to you. Also, share with Him about some of your daily tasks and ask Him to help you accomplish them in a way that brings Him glory. As you continue to practice hearing from God in your personal time and during your sessions with patients, you will be surprised by how quickly they recover from their illnesses and how many adverse events are prevented. I'm not saying that you will never again have another misdiagnosis, but what I am saying is that God has answers that He is ready to give you to more effectively help your patients. Your ability to hear God's direction can literally mean life or death for your patients. Time is of the essence.

Disconnecting from God Is a Two-Edged Sword: It Affects You Too

The consequence for health-care professionals who have disconnected themselves from God is like a two-edged sword. By doing so, they have cut off their ability to hear from the Lord to better treat their patients, and they have also made themselves vulnerable to the same health conditions that they are helping to treat in others. Instead of being equipped, many of them have become susceptible to depression, dementia, anxiety, fear, Parkinson's disease, diabetes, and even cancer. I cannot tell you the number of highly educated individuals I have come across whose purposes in life have been diminished by terminal illnesses. I have served renowned psychologists, medical doctors, scientists, and others with PhDs who were forced to spend their golden years with the same debilitating diseases that they had once been experts in treating. As I saw this on a repeated basis, I was grieved. It hurt me to see them suffering this way, and what was worse was the fact that they spoke without hope. They knew that they would not become better, and they didn't. Some of them died and left their potential in the grave.

Although some of these individuals developed their illnesses in their older years, there are younger ones with habits that they are fighting against and failing miserably. Without God in your life, you have no hope and are forced to face the storms of life alone. There are doctors and nurses who are quick to advise their patients to quit smoking but can't kick the habit themselves. What would motivate a doctor to start smoking cigarettes when he or she has seen what the human lungs look like after years of smoking? Stress. Anxiety. Pressures of life. Nobody is immune from stress, especially in the medical field where people are placed in highly demanding work environments. Sure, many facilities have made significant adjustments to help solve this problem, but these efforts aren't enough. How do you deal with the pressure of performing a critical operation that will impact the rest of your patient's life? Do you rely solely on your antianxiety medication, do you puff up your ego, or do you pray? Do you ask God to touch your hands so that the surgery will turn out successful? These are very practical things that you should be doing if you are in a position of caring for people.

The Inevitable Guilt

Before I leave this topic, I need to address one more aspect of it. The feeling of guilt over a patient's downturn is something that many health professionals experience at one point. Even if the person wasn't directly under your care, you may feel like you could have done more to help him or her. One of Satan's tactics in hindering your effectiveness as a clinician is to convince you that what happened to your patient was your fault. He may say to you, "If only you had tried this …" or "You should not have made that move. It was a big mistake." Satan will attempt to bring you down with these lies, but that's not what God would say to you if you would hear Him. (I say *would* and not *could* because God is always speaking, but without a relationship with Him, you can't hear His voice.) He would whisper gently to your heart and tell you that you did the best you could, and He loves you. He may also share with you several ideas to improve your clinical skills that you may have omitted. Either way, you will experience His peace, love, and comfort even when you feel like a failure. A personal relationship with Jesus is *the* missing piece in health-care practices. Without it, health professionals may lose a sense of their purpose and even become distracted by some of the social issues that arise in a health-care system.

Competition with One Another

I have often been asked why I never worked in a hospital setting. The answer is easy. I was deterred by some of the things that I saw during my clinical rotations as a student. One of the main issues I observed was competition among some of the health-care workers. There were nurses who felt threatened by some of the tasks that the pharmacists were taking on; one area was in counseling patients as they were discharged. At times this conflict arose because one party felt that their responsibilities were being taken away, while the other party didn't feel that their expertise was properly utilized. Also, a few doctors were a little annoyed that some of the pharmacists called themselves "Dr. So and So" (because of their doctorate degrees), and at times, there was a little confusion as to who was what. Finally, some pharmacists felt that they had to prove themselves to be recognized in their work environment. Although there is nothing wrong with wanting your professional skills to be utilized at a maximal level, it must be done for the right reasons. If your goal isn't to work together to help patients become well, then your efforts will be unfruitful.

When I was a pharmacy student, this idea to make our clinical qualifications apparent was ingrained into us daily. I remember during one of my interviews for a pharmacy residence program, I had just finished my presentation and was asked a few questions. One of the questions was, "In what ways can you prove yourself as a professional?" I replied, "By doing what I am trained to do. If I perform my tasks according to my professional training, I prove myself this way. I don't think I necessarily have to do anything extravagant." As you may have guessed, some of the panelists did not like that response, and I didn't match that residency program.

What is the point that I am making here? I am not saying that health-care professionals should not work hard to be qualified or even to show others their qualifications. What

I am saying is that the motive behind everything you do is crucial. Boosting your ego and itching for someone to tell you that "you know your stuff" should never be the driving force to do anything in your professional field. There are people whom the Lord has placed under your care where you work, and it is your duty to work with those around you so that your patients receive optimal health care. This cannot be accomplished if one group is fighting with the other group because their recommendation is not acknowledged. Every task that health professionals accomplish should be done to the glory of God, not for their own glory. The next time you get into a conflict with another member of your medical team, identify the real motive. Purpose to honor the Lord in everything that you do.

Development of Apathy

As a student in a health professional program, you are fed a lot of knowledge, some of which you may forget and some of which you may remember for life. When your schooling was over, you may have felt empowered and ready to save the world, but something happened shortly after that. As you stepped further into your career, you realized that you didn't know enough. You realized that you needed further learning.

I recall an event when I experienced my own limitations as well, not academically but physically. Organic chemistry was one of my favorite subjects because I understood it and excelled in it. I received no less than an A-plus on every exam, and the last course exam was no exception. What was unique about this final exam was that two of my friends also excelled on it. As we gathered around, hugging each other and rejoicing, one of my friends stepped hard on my foot close to my ankle and I fell to the floor. As I got up, I found it difficult to stand on my left foot, and I honestly thought that it was broken. After the school nurse took an x-ray, she concluded that it was sprained and recommended that I wrap it daily and use crutches for some time. This may not be significant to most people, but it was to me. As an athlete at that time, I was used to running on rough surfaces and occasionally twisting an ankle, but I always bounced back quickly. As I walked with crutches for about a week, I realized that I wasn't as invincible as I thought and that I could really get hurt.

The point of this story is to illustrate that you are going to arrive at a point where you come face to face with your own limitations. You can choose to enhance your learning or become apathetic and feel hopeless. The learning that I am referring to isn't just going to a textbook, although this is very important. I am talking about getting wisdom from God instead of just relying on what you know from experience or from your studies. Wisdom is different from knowledge because wisdom is involved in the application of the knowledge that you have. It will show you *how* to use the *what* you already know.

Apathy sometimes develops over time when you see the same event occur over and over in your patients and the end results mirror one another. After years of seeing people perish under the same types of illnesses, it is not unusual for some health professionals to get used to it. Apathy begins to settle in, and it causes them to lose compassion and even the drive to keep helping their patients. As I mentioned above, you are God's agent to minister to your patients, and you fulfill this role by doing your best to help them get well. When familiarity and apathy begin to settle in, go back and recall the reason that you're in your field in the first place. Go to God and ask Him for His wisdom to better serve your patients. Another reason you as a health professional should involve God in your daily practices is to prevent apathy and rekindle the fire that you once had to help your patients.

In conclusion, you are in your field on purpose. You may have thought that you chose your career because someone advised you to do so. However, this is not completely true. Sure, someone may have planted a seed in you, but that drive to meet the needs of people around you came from God. Just as His nature is to bring healing to hurting people, He placed this same nature in you so that you can help a dying world. Although healing takes various forms, the results are similar. Now that you've seen examples of healers in the natural world, allow me to reintroduce you to the original healer.

Chapter 5: God, the Original Healer

The Need for a Healer

With all the natural and synthetic medicine widely available today, you may wonder why there is still a need for a healer. Well, let me ask you a question: Are you cured of the conditions that you're currently taking medications to treat? If your answer is no, then you still need a healer. The healing that I am referring to is not a psychological state of mind or a metaphysical delusion but a real, tangible change in your health condition. According to the *Merriam-Webster Dictionary*, to heal is "to make free from injury or disease: to make sound or whole."[1] It also means "to make well again and to restore whole."

Most of the medications today are not effective enough to restore a person back to good health. They may provide temporary or sustained relief from certain symptoms, but as soon as that medication is discontinued, the body reverts to its original problematic state. Hence, most medications that people take today are considered "maintenance meds." These maintenance medications are used to treat conditions such as high blood pressure, anxiety, depression, arthritis, high cholesterol, pain, asthma, and more. Some medications aid in eliminating certain disease states, but certain factors play into their effectiveness. For example, many antibiotics do help to cure specific types of bacterial infections, but—as you know if you're familiar with how antibiotics work—a good immune system is required for most of them to be efficacious. Antibiotics such as doxycycline, tetracycline, clindamycin, and azithromycin exert their effects by stopping the susceptible bacteria from continuing to replicate until the body's immune system can properly eliminate the bacterial infection. On the other hand, penicillin antibiotics (penicillin, amoxicillin, ampicillin, and more) have the potential to kill the bacteria, but they are not always very effective because of bacterial resistance.

Most of the medications today do a great job in suppressing symptoms but have very little impact on the root cause of those symptoms; therefore, the symptoms often recur once the medication is removed. Many health-care professionals today would have their patients believe that their health conditions are primarily due to poor lifestyle habits (poor diet or insufficient activity level), genetics, environmental factors, poor adherence to their medications, or just a normal process of aging. Most of the counseling that health-care professionals provide their patients is centered on adherence to these medications, and they offer little hope of ever coming off of them. The root cause of a wide range of health problems is not necessarily found in a laboratory result or on a monitoring screen but is often emotional and even spiritual. Please allow me to explain.

Some of the top medical conditions treated today are anxiety or anxiety-related disorders (bulimia, obsessive-compulsive disorder, posttraumatic stress disorder), depression, high blood pressure, and sleep disorders. In the areas of anxiety and depression especially, health-care professionals are gaining a better understanding that these conditions are directly connected to an event or events that have occurred in a person's life. Some people have experienced life-altering, traumatic events during their childhood or adolescence that have led to their disease state. Other people have become sick because of the day-to-day stress of life: stress at work, at home, at school, or due to a broken relationship. High blood pressure is not just caused by having too much salt in your diet but is also linked to prolonged exposure to stressful environments. Many sleep disorders are also related to stress and anxiety.

These examples so far are easily identifiable as anxiety or stress-related, but what about other conditions such as rheumatoid arthritis or infections that have measurable indicators for their diagnoses? What are the root causes of these conditions? The answer lies in John 10:10 (NKJV): "The thief does not come except to steal, and to kill, and to destroy. I have come that they may have life, and that they may have *it* more abundantly." The thief is Satan, the enemy of God and humankind. Don't be spooked by this, but be informed that there is a spiritual being named Satan who, since the beginning of the world, has tried to make people sick and kill them. Every medical condition that you can think of is traced back to him. God, on the other hand, solely desires to heal you and give you an enjoyable life.

Practically speaking, how can any of this be true when it's been proven that certain chemical deficiencies or imbalances cause abnormalities in the body? The answer is in the way that humankind was created. It was mentioned earlier in this book that men and women are three-part beings made up of a spirit, soul, and body (1 Thess. 5:23 KJV). When God created Adam in His own image, He created him a spirit being just like Him. Inside that spirit being, He placed a soul, which comprises the mind, will, and emotions. Last, He created Adam's physical body and put that created spirit in Adam's physical body. The Bible says in Genesis 2:7 (NKJV), "And the Lord God formed man *of* the dust of the ground, and breathed into his nostrils the breath of life; and man became a living being." The "breath of life" is also known as the spirit.

Without going too deep, Satan throws circumstances into people's paths to cause illness in their bodies. In the example of an infection, God created the human body with a natural defense system to fight infections. He created your immune system and barrier methods to prevent diseases. Two of these barrier methods are the skin and mucus membranes, which are found in the eyes, oral cavity, and other parts of the body. He also designed you with a healthy, normal bacterial flora on your skin, mouth, and other open cavities of the body to prevent certain types of infections from occurring. An infection occurs when there is an overgrowth of certain bacterial organisms or when a foreign organism breaches the body's natural barriers and enters the body. One of Satan's tactics is to bring circumstances into your life that place you under such emotional stress that your immune system is weakened. He often uses people, although they don't realize it, to speak harshly to you, or he may frighten you with the scare of an epidemic. Fear and stress both weaken the body's natural defenses, and since certain infections occur because of a weakened immune system, it's easy to see how many diseases are emotionally and spiritually related.

As for the abnormal lab results that are associated with certain health conditions, they are simply physical manifestations of what has occurred internally. When your emotions (the soul part of you) are experiencing stress, your body reflects that stress by releasing a hormone called cortisol.[2] In an urgent situation, cortisol is necessary because it allows you to be alert and focused, especially in the event of danger. Prolonged emotional stress, however, causes higher levels of cortisol to be present, which can raise blood sugar and blood pressure, hinder the ability to form strong bones, and more. Also, when you are under prolonged stress, an imbalance may occur between norepinephrine (an adrenaline hormone) and serotonin (a sleep chemical), resulting in insomnia or depressive symptoms. Additionally, chronic anger, bitterness, and unforgiveness, which are associated with negative emotions, may increase the likelihood of heart disease, diabetes, hypertension, and more.[3] The emotional part of human beings is where Satan often attacks in order to create abnormalities in their bodies. God desires to provide you with a solid defense mechanism to prevent illnesses from occurring in your mind and body.

Jesus Christ, the Healer

Many people all over the world have heard about Jesus Christ but have very little understanding of who He really is or what He came to do while He was on the earth. Some institutions lump Him with other philosophers or religious teachers and don't see anything unique about Him. Jesus Christ is unlike any other philosopher, prophet, or religious teacher who has ever existed. He isn't just God's representative, like many of the other prophets in the Bible; He is the Son of God and God Himself. In John 8:42 (NKJV), Jesus described where He came from originally. He said, "I proceeded forth and came from God; nor have I come of Myself, but He sent Me." He reiterated this statement again in the sixteenth chapter.

Jesus came to exist on the earth through a supernatural working of the Holy Spirit and was born of a virgin girl named Mary. Although He walked, talked, and looked like a man, He had a divine nature. In John 8:56 (NKJV), Jesus told the religious leaders of the day, "Your father Abraham rejoiced to see My day, and he saw *it* and was glad." He made this statement to reveal to His audience (the Jews) that Abraham, who had been dead for thousands of years, saw Him leave heaven and come down to the earth, and he rejoiced over it. Then His audience replied with, "You are not yet fifty years old, and have You seen Abraham?" Jesus answered, "Most assuredly, I say to you, before Abraham was, I AM." To fully grasp the impact of Jesus's claim to be "I AM" or God, you must refer to where this statement originated.

In Exodus 3, God appeared to Moses and told him to go back to Egypt, where he initially grew up, to deliver His people (the Israelites) from the bondage of slavery and oppression. In verse 13, Moses asked God to tell him His name, and God replied, "'I AM WHO I AM' … thus you shall say to the children of Israel, 'I AM has sent me to you'" (Exo. 3:14 NKJV). Furthermore, God said, "Thus you shall say to the children of Israel: 'The LORD God of your fathers, the God of Abraham, the God of Isaac, and the God of Jacob, has sent me to you. This *is* My name forever, and this *is* My memorial to all generations'" (Exo. 3:15 NKJV). The name "I AM" is God's eternal name, revealing that He was in the past, is in the present, and will be in the future. He can stand in any position of time and see what has happened, what is happening, and what is going to happen.

This is the reason He could reveal to the prophets of the Old and New Testaments things that pertained to Israel's past and current spiritual climate, as well as the church's.

Jesus also bears that same title. We see another example of it in the book of Revelation. Jesus said to John, "I *am* He who lives, and was dead, and behold, I am alive forevermore" (Rev. 1:18 NKJV). You may read this verse and become a little confused because it doesn't make sense to the natural mind. If you will allow me to, I will clarify. Jesus's existence did not begin on the earth. In fact, He has no beginning or ending. The pictures that you see of Him when you step into churches are portraits of His physical body after He was born on the earth. He is not a created being like God's angels, animals, man, or any form of matter. He is the physical representation of God in appearance and character. When you have an encounter with Jesus, you have also had an encounter with God Himself.

Like the people of Jesus's day, many individuals today often struggle with some of Jesus's teachings. For those who haven't been informed, Jesus is the Savior, healer, and restorer of humanity. He came to eliminate the distance between God and humankind, which sin had created, and to restore humankind back to the God who loved and cared for them. Jesus sums up His entire purpose for coming to the earth in John 3:16 (NKJV): "For God so loved the world that He gave His only begotten Son, that whoever believes in Him should not perish but have everlasting life." To access this everlasting life, all you must do is believe in your heart that God raised Jesus from the dead and say with your mouth, "Jesus Christ is Lord. Jesus be the Lord of my life" (Rom. 10:9–10 NKJV). This everlasting life is multifaceted, but I will touch on a few aspects of it. Some aspects of this eternal life include salvation from sin to become in right standing with God, salvation from poverty to become a partaker of the abundant resources of God, and salvation from sickness and disease to become whole again.

Jesus Christ came to bring healing and restoration to the three components of humankind: the spirit, soul, and body. Everything necessary for your wholeness was accomplished at the cross. When Jesus died on the cross, His blood was shed for every area of human life. Some of you have heard of the blood of Jesus but don't understand what it represents. It represents the life of Jesus. Leviticus 17:11 (NKJV) states, "For the life of the flesh *is* in the blood." Naturally speaking, when the blood of a human being stops flowing, death is imminent. Blood is a sign of life. Colossians 1:14 (NKJV) states this about Jesus: "In whom we have redemption through His blood, the forgiveness of sins." In simple terms, the life of Jesus that was in His blood cleansed you of all sin (past, present, and future) the moment that you accepted Him as your Lord and Savior. Do you know something else that is exciting? When He became your Lord and Savior, His life came into you.

Although it's hard for the human mind to conceive this, spiritually speaking, His blood flows in your blood (because His life flows in you). If you have been diagnosed with a blood or bleeding disorder, there is great hope for you. Just as there was no abnormality in Jesus's blood, there ought to be no abnormality in your blood. The key to accessing what Jesus has already paid for through His blood is learning how to apply healing scriptures in the Bible. Jesus's blood will forever impact the human spirit, soul, and body.

If you have an authentic relationship with Jesus Christ, then a healing miracle has taken place in your spirit being. God has blotted out every mistake and every sin that you've ever committed and stripped Satan of the power that he once had over you. To those who believe in Jesus, God says this about you: "Then I will give them one heart, and I will put a new spirit within them, and take the stony heart out of their flesh, and give them a heart of flesh, that they may walk in My statutes and keep My judgments and do them; and they shall be My people, and I will be their God (Ezek. 11:19–20 NKJV). The apostle Paul corroborates this in 2 Corinthians 5:17 (NKJV): "Therefore, if anyone *is* in Christ, *he is* a new creation; old things have passed away; behold, all things have become new." If you're a believer in Jesus Christ, God has removed your previously hard heart (spirit) toward Him and recreated your heart to love Him and follow Him. In this sense, healing has taken place in your spirit. However, God didn't just stop there. He has also made it possible for your soul and body to be completely transformed by the power of God in the name of Jesus.

The soul has often been confused with the spirit, but the two are totally separate, although they are connected to each other. Paul writes in Hebrews 4:12 (NKJV), "For the word of God *is* living and powerful, and sharper than any two-edged sword, piercing even *to the division of soul and spirit, and of joints and marrow*, and is a discerner of the thoughts and intents of the heart" (emphasis added). Just as a joint connects one bone to another bone, the soul is connected to the spirit as well as to the physical body. Your spirit is known as the "hidden person of the heart" (1 Peter 3:4 NKJV) because it's the innermost part of you.

You may be reading this part of the book with questions in your mind. You may ask yourself, *What is the proof that I have a soul or spirit or both?* If you're like me and enjoy watching a good, mushy romance film, you may be able to understand the following illustration. In a typical film, a handsome man meets a beautiful woman, who is usually a little rude to him at first, and falls in love with her (or vice versa). The two eventually hit it off and begin seeing each other. Then, the man or woman becomes afraid that the romance is too good to be true, or hurts from the past may come up. Either way, one party or both run away. As they seek counsel from their friends, do you know what advice is usually given? It is this: "Follow your heart." If the couple had fallen in love and developed feelings for each other, why did they back out of the relationship? They did so because there was an internal conflict; a part of them had deep emotions for the other person, while the other part of them was focusing on the potential downfall of the relationship. When you are told in movies to follow your heart, it implies that there is a difference between what you are thinking or feeling and what your heart is telling you to do. What you're thinking or feeling is the soul part of you, and what your heart is telling you is what your spirit is telling you. This is easy to see, isn't it?

As stated earlier, your soul is made up of your mind, will, and emotions. One of the areas in which many people today suffer is in their emotions. Fear, anxiety, depression, worry, hatred, bitterness, and jealousy have had such a lasting grip on numerous individuals that they are sick mentally and even physically. As also stated before, fear, anxiety, and depression are the top three emotion-related conditions that are treated today. In fact, it's become normal to prescribe medications for anxiety such as clonazepam, diazepam, lorazepam, fluoxetine, and others. Diagnoses of depression are being made at an ever-increasing rate, and antidepressants are being prescribed for depressed mood caused by loss of family members, loss of job, tragedy, traumatic events, and other situations. So many people are overwhelmed with the distresses of life that they feel hopeless and believe that medicine is their only hope. What's more troubling is that anxiety and depression don't just affect adults; little children experience these symptoms as well. Although antidepressants have other indications besides anxiety and depressed states, these are the reasons that they are prescribed most of the time. These medications often provide some relief, but as I mentioned before, they belong to the category of maintenance meds.

Many of these patients are on anxiety medications for years, and some never come off them. This is because the root cause of their symptoms is not properly dealt with. Sure, there is counseling, but counseling without God's help simply rehashes the situation and often leaves the wound feeling fresh again. Psychotherapy and shock therapy have limitations as well. Psychotherapy helps you rationalize and come up with different strategies of thinking, but people often revert to their original state. Shock therapy, which is sometimes used in the most challenging and hard-to-treat cases of mental disorders, only provides temporary relief of symptoms.

God designed humanity to live by every word that He has ever spoken. The Bible is the bread that you are to feed on to receive daily nourishment of your spirit, which impacts your soul and body. What does it mean to live by every word of God? It's reading and meditating on it daily and doing what it instructs you to do. It's believing what it says and applying it to every area of your life.

When you consider it, this isn't a strange thing to say. Think about the songs that you're faithful to learn or the sports event you're faithful to attend or watch. You've probably never missed a game of your favorite sports team. I am often amazed at how fanatics can quote every play or score that their team has achieved. Despite my athletic background,

I have never been a real fan of sports, compared to other people I know. However, what interests me is music. When I was in my early teens, MTV had this show called *Total Request Live* (I believe it still airs today). Every day, I faithfully turned on the television, flipped to the station, and watched the music videos that made the top ten or twenty list. I lived by every song, reciting every lyric in my head and dancing along. I memorized lyrics to songs by Britney Spears, Christina Aguilera, Mandy Moore, Backstreet Boys, NSYNC, and more. Just as a teenager or young child can be addicted to lyrics, humankind can be addicted to the words that God speaks, both the written and the spoken words that He speaks to their heart. In fact, you were created for this exact purpose.

Instead of turning to God, men and women have turned to talk show hosts or tabloid magazines and are left empty, sick, lonely, and brokenhearted. God created you to have fellowship with Him and sent Jesus to be the healer of your emotions. Jesus says in Matthew 11:28–30 NKJV, "Come to Me, all *you* who labor and are heavy laden, and I will give you rest." If you suffer from terrible anxiety, Jesus longs to give you rest. He desires to fill your heart and mind with His peace. He is strong and powerful enough to remove the stronghold in your mind that keeps you in a depressed state. Depression was not created by God, and therefore, He sent Jesus to deliver you from it. Jesus died on the cross to deliver His people from toxic emotions that have led to many of the mental disorders seen today. Healing from anxiety, depression, hatred, or anger is sometimes a gradual process, but Jesus specializes in these areas and can bring complete healing to the soul.

When internal issues are not dealt with but are left unresolved, these problems often manifest as a sickness or disease in the body. There are people today who have allowed bitterness to fester deep inside their hearts so that their bodies are frail, tired, and worn out. While on the subject, bitterness is an emotion that you must guard against daily. It is easy for it to develop toward co-workers and family members—especially family members. Being overly critical of others is the door to developing bitterness. In one of the stores where I worked, there was a young lady who was so mean to those around her, even to her supervisors (which I didn't understand because they had the power to fire her). Every time I walked into the store and saw her, I groaned silently because of the treatment I knew I would receive from her. I cannot exaggerate about how nasty she was, but do you know why she was that way? She was frustrated at the financial and emotional circumstances that she faced. As she continued this way for a few years, she developed a life-threatening illness. She eventually recovered from it and became a little nicer. The point that I am making is that persistent bitterness, anger, and other toxic emotions must be resolved quickly. Otherwise, they can cost someone his or her life.

While bitterness and other negative emotions play a role in the development of illness, they are also responsible for wreaking havoc in the body. Many heart-related conditions are due to these emotions. I mentioned during my introduction that I had experienced some tightening in my chest during my early days as a pharmacist because of my stressful work environment. Others in my field have developed high blood pressure due to the rigorous daily requirements. I recall that, not too long ago, a former colleague of mine had been feeling more and more anxious at work and began to take medication to help her symptoms. She continued to work hard to accomplish daily responsibilities despite being short-staffed almost daily. She began to develop heart palpitations because of persistent stress. Things grew worse to the point that, one day, she closed her pharmacy early and went to the emergency room to have her heart evaluated. I shared this true story so that you may know that there are people who can identify with your current situation.

Although some of these soul issues will have to be dealt with to achieve full recovery, Jesus can heal your physical body even in the state that you are currently if you'll allow Him to. Acts 10:38 (NKJV) says that "God anointed Jesus of Nazareth with the Holy Spirit and with power, who went about doing good and healing all who were oppressed by the devil, for God was with Him." This healing included the blind recovering their sight, the lame walking, lepers' being cleansed, deaf ears opening, and people being raised from the dead (Luke 7:22 KJV). Jesus is also able to heal health problems other than these. The Bible says in Galatians 3:13 (KJV) that "Christ redeemed us from the curse of the Law … that the blessing of Abraham might come on the Gentiles through Jesus Christ." The curse of law included inflammatory conditions, fever, consumption or tuberculosis, plaques or epidemics (bacterial or viral), sores, chronic illnesses, and more. Jesus can heal you of any acute or chronic illness that you may be experiencing.

Any healing that you will ever receive from God comes through Jesus alone. Jesus is not just *able* to heal you; He is also *willing* to heal you. True healing comes from two sources: God's Word and God's presence. The first way to receive your healing is to spend time reading the Bible and identifying healing scriptures, meditating on those scriptures until you believe them with your heart, and declaring with your mouth what you believe God will heal you from. Another way to receive healing is listening to someone teach you those healing scriptures, and a third way is to spend time in God's presence, in praising and worshipping Him. The next chapter will elaborate further on how to receive your healing using these methods.

Chapter 6: Where True Healing Comes From

God's Word Is the True Medicine

Although millions of people all over the world have criticized the Bible and concluded that its contents are myths or fairy tales, this is far from true. The same God who created plants and microbial organisms, from which many medications have been derived, has provided a collection of books from which healing can be obtained. Contrary to some of the teachings today about the Bible, the Bible was written by people who were moved by the Spirit of God. In 2 Timothy 3:16 in the New International Version, we find, "All Scripture is God-breathed and is useful for teaching, rebuking, correcting and training in righteousness, so that the servant of God may be thoroughly equipped for every good work." Simply put, every word in the Bible is a reliable source to teach, train, correct, and equip you for whatever you need. Hebrews 9:8 (NLT) identifies the Holy Spirit as the true author of Scripture, not mere men. Paul makes the following statement in this passage: "the Holy Spirit revealed...."

In the previous chapter, I used the term "God's DNA" but reserved its true explanation until now. To illustrate the fact that the words of the Bible came from God and contain the power and nature of God, I will do so in natural terms. The Word of God is referred to as incorruptible seed, and each "word" or seed contains the DNA of God or the divine nature of God to bring what that word is saying to pass. When you asked Jesus to be your Lord and Savior, you obtained those words from Romans 10:9–10. When you verbalized them, the seeds of those words entered your heart, subsequently causing you to be born again and allowing Jesus to come into your heart in the form of the Holy Spirit. Jesus is the Word of God, and "all things were made by Him; and without Him was not anything made that was made" (John 1:1 KJV).

Do you know whom you are staring at every time you read the Bible? Jesus. By moving upon people to write the words of the Bible, the Holy Spirit revealed Jesus and the character of God in every verse. In John 16:13–15 (NKJV), Jesus tells His disciples, "However, when He, the Spirit of truth, has come, He will guide you into all truth.… He will take of what is Mine and declare *it* to you." The words of Scripture can produce results when they are believed and acted upon because there is a person (Jesus Christ) behind those words who is being revealed.

Going back to the seed illustration, there is another aspect of the Word of God as seed to be mentioned. Unlike a variety of seeds, which are needed to grow different types of fruits such as apples, oranges, and grapes, there is only one seed source (Jesus) in the Bible. However, each of the different passages of Scripture can produce a variety of results. Every word of Scripture contains the essence or life of Jesus, thereby revealing different aspects of the nature of God. The nature of God is infinitely diverse. One aspect of His nature is the fruit that He bears, which is "love, joy, peace, longsuffering (patience), kindness, goodness, faithfulness, gentleness, self-control" (Gal. 5:22–23 NKJV). Another aspect of His nature that is revealed in the words of Scripture is His healing power. In fact, the words of the Bible are analogous to medicine that is used to treat health problems in the body. Proverbs 4:20–22 (NKJV) states, "My son, give attention to my words; incline your ear to my sayings. Do not let them depart from your eyes; keep them in the midst of your heart; for they *are* life to those who find them, and health to all their flesh." If you have a King James Bible, the cross-reference replaces the word *health* with *medicine.* How is the Word of God analogous to medicine? It produces the same effect in the body. When a medication is taken by mouth or injected into the veins, it eventually travels to the site where it is needed. Unless you are observed with a probe, you as the patient don't comprehend how it travels throughout the body and relieves your symptoms, nor do you need to know. All that is important is that the medicine helps you feel better. This is the same way with the Word of God. When you read it, hear it, meditate on it, or speak it, you don't know exactly how it's going to work. However, what happens is that the power of God is released, and it goes straight to the area where it is needed.

I have countless stories that I could share about the application of God's Word and its effect in the body, but I will limit it to one. In one of the stores where I traveled to work, one of the front-end staff members who was helping at the pharmacy shared with me that her husband was very ill and had been hospitalized for a while. She also shared that after her daily shifts, she went to visit him and sat by his bedside until visiting hours ended. As a doctor prescribes medicine to be taken for relief of symptoms, I wrote down on a piece of paper a few scriptures and advised her to read them to her husband daily. After my shift was over, I left that store and returned a few weeks later. When I saw this young woman again, I had totally forgotten about what I had shared with her a few weeks earlier. She came up to me, gave me a hug, and said that she had done what I recommended and noticed significant improvements in her husband's condition. She mentioned that he was able to get up and move around, which he couldn't do before. I encouraged her to continue to read the verses to her husband until he experienced full recovery.

When you read the healing scriptures that are provided at the end of this book, it is not important to try to figure out how they will affect your body. All that is necessary to know is that as you read them, God's power is released into your body and will work without any negative side effects.

It has always been God's will for His people to receive the healing benefits of His Word. Therefore, He told the Israelites in Deuteronomy 7:12–15 (NKJV) that if they would keep His commandments (His Word), He would take away from them "all sickness and will put none of the terrible diseases of Egypt" upon them. The medicinal or healing power of God, which pervades all of Scripture, can have tremendous impact in areas often overlooked. In the above passage of Deuteronomy, God also promises to "bless the fruit of your womb," which applies to those of you who need a healing in your infertile womb. Maybe you don't need a healing in your body today, but you may need a healing in failing areas of your business. If you are a farmer and your livelihood depend on the crops that are produced or on the animals that you possess, God promises to heal your land so that your crops can yield great harvest and your animals can continue to multiply. If farming is not your forte but you have certain goals and dreams you wish to accomplish, He provides the following instructions in Joshua 1:8 (NKJV) to be successful: "This Book of the Law shall not depart from your mouth, but you shall meditate in it day and night, that you may observe to do according to all that is written in it. For then you will make your way prosperous, and then you will have good success." Throughout the centuries, many people have thought of God's commandments as burdensome, but that was not His intent. His intent was to provide you a thorough list of parameters within which to walk so that you would have access to His healing virtues and live healed, financially prosperous, and abounding with joy.

The Bible is full of the healing power of God and so versatile that the same passage of scripture can produce joy and peace during times of depression and sadness while empowering you with ideas and concepts to have a successful and prosperous business. Using Joshua 1:8 as an example, God's Word can fill your heart with the hope that He has the answer you need to be successful, which consequently stirs up joy inside of you while your restless heart becomes at peace. As you continue to meditate on that verse and other related verses, He will begin to give you ideas and strategies that you haven't thought of.

Please allow me to reiterate that none of what I am saying is fictitious; I live this out every single day. On a consistent basis, God gives me brilliant ideas within just a few hours of meditating on His Word and spending time in prayer. To receive whatever you need from God, whether it's healing in your body, healing in your mind, or strategies to overcome difficult circumstances, the process is the same. Proverbs 4:20–22 and Joshua 1:8 provide the basic formula: constantly reading the Word (keeping it before your eyes), hearing it (listening to it), meditating on it (retaining it in your heart), and speaking it out loud.

You may be wondering how to constantly spend time reading the Word with your busy schedule. I recommend getting up a little earlier before you leave your home to go to work. One practical thing that I did was to write one or two verses of scripture on a small sheet of paper and carry it around with me. I read them silently as I performed my daily tasks at work, and instead of hindering my work, it improved it. I was more focused, less stressed, and provided better customer service than before. I also made fewer mistakes and caught errors much more quickly. You may say, "How?" The more you spend time with God, the more you can hear Him speak to you about things pertaining to your life, including your job. When you develop a greater hunger for Him, He will satisfy that hunger.

In the upcoming chapters, I will provide greater detail on how to practically apply the above formula in everyday living. For now, there is yet another important source from which God's healing can be obtained. Out of the words of the Bible, as well as in His presence, flow His healing attributes.

The Presence of God

You may read this section and wonder why I first discussed the Word of God as the primary source of healing followed by the actual presence of God. Even though healing flows from His manifested presence, without the Bible as your primary reference for how to enter the presence of God, your spiritual experience isn't authentic but could very well be a false substitute. Many individuals have had spiritual experiences with reading materials other than Scripture, but the spiritual power that they plug into by doing so is not of God—it is a false idol. When you enter the presence of God, the Father, the Son, and the Holy Spirit are in your midst.

How do you enter the presence of God? You enter it by praising and worshipping Him. Psalm 22:3 in the Amplified Bible Classic Edition states the following: "But You are holy, O You Who dwell in [the holy place where] the praises of Israel [are offered]." The New King James Version translates this passage as follows: "But You *are* holy, enthroned in the praises of Israel." In the Old Testament, before Jesus was on the earth, the place of worship where people could go to offer sacrifices, praises, and worship to God was in the temple of God, which was originally built by King Solomon (really, under his leadership) and then later rebuilt after it was destroyed. When Jesus began His earthly ministry, He introduced the true desire of God where worship was concerned: that God wasn't looking for a mere building but was looking for people with a genuine heart to worship Him. In John 4:23 (NKJV), Jesus replies to a question asked by a woman regarding the location of worship. He said, "But the hour is coming, and now is, when the true worshipers will worship the Father *in spirit and truth; for the Father is seeking such to worship Him"* (emphasis added).

If you're like I was, you may be wondering why God desires to be worshipped. Is it so that His ego can be stoked? No. On the contrary, He desires your worship so that He can be close to you. He desires to be the object of your focus instead of other earthly things. What does it mean to worship something? It is to ascribe reverence, awe, honor, and praise to that thing. It also means to prostrate yourself before an object or person or to place yourself under the influence of a thing. Whether you realize it or not, everyone has an object of worship. For some it's God, but for others it's a statue of an idol such as Buddha. For many, their object of worship may be someone with great academic accomplishments or a famous Hollywood star. Does this sound familiar to you? Many of you have watched the show *American Idol,* but have you ever stopped to think about what the title really means? Sure, it's a great show that seeks out and develops upcoming singing talent. However, when you observe the title closely with respect to the content of the show, you realize that the program is designed to create the next "star" to be emulated or looked up to. I am not saying that it is wrong to think very highly of people. In fact, you should. What I am saying is that there are objects or people that you worship without even realizing it. Anything that you hold in honor, respect, or adoration above God is considered an idol.

Going back to why God desires to be worshipped, He seeks it for several reasons. First, He longs to draw close to you and reveal Himself to you. He desires an avenue by which He can connect to humankind, and worship is one of the ways that this is accomplished. Second, He yearns to be the object of your focus, not the material things of this world. There ought not to be anything that comes between you and the Lord. He understands that you have other responsibilities such as a family to take care of and a career to build, but He should be your priority. He wants you to look to Him for help first when you're in trouble, not anyone else. He longs to be the best friend with whom you share intimate secrets. Third, He desires for you to enjoy the pleasure of His presence. Worship is intimate by nature and allows you to draw close to the heart of God so that you may hear from Him. Before I continue, allow me to delve deeper into the functions of praise and worship and how they are intertwined.

Praise and Worship

You may be asking yourself, *How do I praise and worship God?* Although both are closely related and go hand in hand, there are a few differences that I will point out. Praise affirms God's creation and His mighty acts, and it is typically based on what He has done for an individual. An illustration of this can be found in Psalm 150:1–2 (NKJV): "Praise God in His sanctuary; praise Him in His mighty firmament! praise Him for His mighty acts; praise Him according to His excellent greatness!" Another example is found in Exodus 15:2 (NKJV), which states, "The Lord *is* my strength and song, and He has become my salvation; He *is* my God, and I will praise Him; my father's God, and I will exalt Him." In fact, many of the chapters in the book of Psalms are about praising God and provide great insight on how praises are offered to Him. It's not surprising that many of the contemporary Christian songs today are based on the book of Psalms.

Furthermore, praises aren't offered with words alone but are accompanied with expressions. Praises are offered with the clapping of hands, shouting, dancing, playing of instruments, and much more. An example is found in Psalm 47:1 (NKJV): "Oh, clap your hands, all you peoples! Shout to God with the voice of triumph!" You may have attended a church service where people were dancing and clapping their hands and thought to yourself, *What are they doing?* What they were doing was praising God! I enjoy attending churches of other denominations to observe the different styles of services. In some places, the people are very solemn and hardly smile, while in other places, they can't sit still very long. For those of you who thought that praising God ought to be done quietly, you thought wrong. Psalm 150:4–6 (NKJV) states, "Praise Him with the timbrel and *dance*; Praise Him with stringed instruments and flutes! Praise Him with *loud* cymbals; Praise Him with *clashing* cymbals! Let everything that has breath praise the LORD. Praise the LORD!" (emphasis added). When you come before God, there ought to be freedom to express your love for Him. Allow yourself to dance before Him like King David in the Bible did, and don't be afraid of what people think. God isn't ashamed of you, so don't be ashamed of Him!

While praise typically affirms God's loving actions toward humanity, worship, on the other hand, typically affirms His divine nature and divine attributes. In other words, worship is centered on *who* He is and not just on *what* He has done. An illustration of this is found in Psalm 29:2 (NKJV), which states, "Give unto the Lord the *glory due to His name*; worship the Lord in the beauty of holiness" (emphasis added). Another example of this is in Psalm 99:5 (NKJV): "Exalt the Lord our God, and worship at His footstool—He *is* holy." Unlike praise, which is accompanied with a variety of expressions, worship has two primary expressions: kneeling down, bowing down, or both. Genesis 24:26 (NKJV) states, "Then the man *bowed down his head* and *worshiped* the Lord" (emphasis added). In Psalm 95:6 (NKJV), both expressions are present: "Oh come, let us worship and *bow down*; let us *kneel* before the Lord our Maker" (emphasis added).

As mentioned above, praise and worship are the major avenues to entering the authentic presence of God. If you are just finding out about this and would like to know where to start, begin with the book of Psalms. As you cultivate a relationship with the Lord and begin to know Him better, praise will be birthed out of your own experiences with Him. As your health improves or difficult circumstances are resolved, you'll have your own unique expression of praise because of a thankful heart. You see, the great thing about praise is that there is general praise, which touches on God's creation, and there is also individual praise, which is expressed out of a personal experience with the Lord. As a beginner, a practical way to praise Him is thanking Him for the things that you currently have—your family, job, home, business, and more. Spend time daily reflecting on His goodness toward you, and praises will flow out of it. The more you experience God's healing power over your mind, body, family, or possessions, the more your "praise vocabulary" will expand. You then begin to thank Him for being your healer, your provider, your protector, and so on.

When you take the next step and begin to worship Him, then you can step into a higher dimension of the presence of God. When you worship Him, He comes in your midst because He has been waiting there all along for you. You don't to have years of experience to worship God. As mentioned before, praise and worship often go hand in hand. Because worship involves intimacy with God (no, not sexual), it's often easier to start out with praise to get your mind focused on the goodness of God. As you praise further, you begin to get a sense of how great and majestic He is and can easily transition into worship. To worship Him, simply kneel or bow down and acknowledge Him. Just as there is individual praise, there is also individual worship, in which you focus on His divine attributes (His majesty, splendor, holiness) but also on Him as healer, redeemer, Savior, and more. Sometimes the fine line between praise and worship becomes hazy because the two operate together in a continuous flow.

Living in a society where individuals have a variety of spiritual experiences, you may ask yourself, *How do I know that what I am experiencing during praise and worship is really from God and authentic?* The presence of God is marked by tremendous joy, peace, healing, restoration, deliverance, revelation knowledge, and more. When you're in His presence, you will experience laughter, rest, strength, a feeling of being refreshed, hope, and most importantly, love because God is love (1 John 4:16 KJV). Psalm 16:11 (NKJV) states, "You will show me the path of life; *in Your presence is fullness of joy*; At Your right hand *are pleasures forevermore*" (emphasis added). In other words, when you get close to God, His "aura" is joy such as you've never experienced. I mentioned earlier about the fruit of the Spirit in Galatians 5:22 (love, joy, peace, patience, gentleness, goodness, faith, meekness, self-control). Notice that love, joy, and peace are also mentioned above and are present when God manifests His presence to His people.

It's not that God simply has these characteristics on the inside of Him; He is full of these traits, but they also *radiate* out of Him. Like a lightbulb radiates light energy, so God radiates the "energy" of joy, love, peace, laughter, and more. Therefore, in Revelation 21:4–5 (KJV), God declares that there will be "no death, neither sorrow, nor crying, neither shall there be any more pain" and that "there shall be no night there; and they need no candle, neither light of the sun; for the Lord God giveth them light." Notice that the above passages describe an environment of no sorrow, darkness, pain, heartache, grief, or tears. When you're around Jesus, the pain of your past leaves and is replaced with hope for the future. Loneliness is replaced with His comfort of love, and sadness gives way to laughter.

Can you now see that when you are in His presence as you praise and worship Him, joy is inevitable? And do you now realize that God can heal your pain-stricken body in just a few minutes of spending time with Him?

Furthermore, the Bible says, "The joy of the LORD is your strength" (Neh. 8:10 NKJV). If you're feeling depressed, anxious, weak, or lonely or are in a difficult predicament, get into the presence of God. Meditate on the book of Psalms, which provides examples on how to offer praises to God during difficult circumstances. Worship God and allow Him to envelop you with the healing power of His love that flows out of Him.

I can personally attest to what I am writing about. There have been days when I've woken up and felt extremely fatigued—so exhausted that I could barely keep my eyes open. When I began to worship the Lord, however, God's presence quickened my body, and I became fully alert and energetic. For a long period of time, I was heartbroken over an individual, but my emotions were usually under control. However, on one day, I woke up feeling a mixture of anger, hurt, pain, and disappointment. I got on my knees and began to thank the Lord for how good He was and is. I told Him how special He was to me and how much I really loved Him. Then I began to worship Him, affirming His majesty, His beauty, and His strength. Sometimes, God gives me new songs during those moments, and He did so on this day. I began to sing the songs, and within a short period of time (less than one hour), I was totally healed of those symptoms.

What I have shared with you is not a psychological experience but a tangible, real-life experience. I'm not speaking based on books that I've read or what others have said; what I am sharing has been birthed out of my walking with the Lord for almost two decades. True healing comes from knowing God in His Word and in His presence. You cannot know Him apart from His Word. If you try to know Him some other way, you will become involved in spiritual things that are real, yes, but are not of God and will eventually destroy your life.

Some individuals may hear about certain people who do healing rituals to help with infertility, for example, and may be curious about them. Your litmus test to determine whether these "healing" practices are safe to participate in is the following: First, are they based on the principles and the teachings of the Bible, or do they contradict them? Second, is Jesus Christ the source of that healing, or is another religious entity mentioned? Third, do these practices require you to perform activities that seem odd? I mention this because, in some groups, animal sacrifices, human sacrifices, or the cutting of human flesh is required. Other odd activities that you should watch out for are the repeating of incantations and spells. Without going deeper into this, understand that for everything that is real, there is a phony substitute that attempts to copy it. The only safeguard against these subtle, crafty practices is the Bible. Authentic and sustained healing comes from spending time reading the Word, particularly healing scriptures, and spending time with God in praise and worship.

Now that you've been enlightened about God being the original creator of medicine and that from His Word and His presence flow healing power, it's time to identify how the two categories (God and medicine) can be merged. In the next chapter, I will illustrate how modern medicine can be combined with the Word of God to achieve remarkable results. I will go even further and say that many of you will eventually arrive at a point where you no longer need to be medicated because the power of God will so affect your body.

Chapter 7: Combining Modern Medicine and the Word of God

Start Where You Are

Applying the teachings of the Bible in your daily life is not only recommended if you want to improve your health; it's a must if you want to see real results. As I mentioned in previous chapters, medicine alone is not effective in curing all your symptoms, particularly in the case of chronic illness. Healing scriptures from the Bible are necessary to greatly improve your health, and they have the potential to bring you to full recovery. In this section, I will provide the practical application of the Word of God in your daily life so that you may be able to apply it to any situation that you encounter.

To begin, it's important to realize that everyone's process of healing is different: some individuals may notice immediate results, while for others, healing is gradual. One of the biggest mistakes that people often make is comparing their results with those of others. You may hear that your neighbor's arthritis completely went away after applying the principles that are taught in this book, and you may be wondering why your symptoms are still hanging around. You must be fully assured that God is no respecter of persons. He is partial to no one and doesn't heal one person and overlook another just because He feels like it. What God is looking for in everyone's heart is faith—not just faith in the head, but faith in the heart. Faith in God, using the name of Jesus, is what moves Him to heal you. Hebrews 11:6 (NLT) says this: "And it is impossible to please God without faith. Anyone who wants to come to him must believe that God exists and that he rewards those who sincerely seek him." In other words, when you ask God to heal you, the only requirements are your believing that He is there and that He will grant your request.

You may ask, *What is faith in God, and how can I obtain it?* Faith in God is simply believing in God's ability to do what He has promised in His Word that He will do. You may also ask yourself, *How can I be so sure that God still heals today?* You can rest assured that God still heals today because He never changes. One of God's missions in sending Jesus Christ on the earth was to make healing available to you. Acts 10:38 (NKJV) states, "God anointed Jesus of Nazareth with the Holy Spirit and with power, who went about doing good and healing all who were oppressed by the devil, for God was with Him." Jesus, who is still alive today, has never stopped fulfilling the Father's assignment for Him. Hebrews 13:8 (NKJV) says that "Jesus Christ *is* the same yesterday, today, and forever." Developing faith in God is necessary to receive anything from Him—healing in your body, mind, family, finances, and more.

How to Develop Faith in God

Just as you develop faith in a person by spending quality time with him or her, so it is with God. You develop faith in Him by reading, meditating, and hearing about His character and His acts in the Bible. As you read in Scripture about the miracles that Jesus performed or those that His disciples performed in Jesus's name, your faith will begin to grow. I want to interject the following statement because I perceive that it is necessary to help your understanding. Many people still do not comprehend why the name of Jesus is being used, so let me explain. God the Father gave Jesus authority over everything that pertains to heaven, earth, and hell. In other words, the name of Jesus carries tremendous weight with the Father and is the only name that He has authorized by which humankind can approach Him and receive from Him. Philippians 2:9–11 (NKJV) states the following: "Therefore God also has highly exalted Him and given Him the name which is above every name, that at the name of Jesus every knee should bow, of those in heaven, and of those on earth, and of those under the earth, and *that* every tongue should confess that Jesus Christ *is* Lord, to the glory of God the Father." Having said this, let's look at two of the miracles that are described in the Bible and observe how they were achieved. Notice how vital faith in God is to receive healing.

The first example comes from the fifth chapter of the book of Mark. A certain woman had suffered from a bleeding disorder for twelve years. Because her chronic condition forced her to seek the help of various physicians, all her finances were eventually depleted. As her condition grew worse, she heard from somewhere that Jesus was in town. Although it was a violation of Jewish law for her to be out in public in her condition, she risked her life because she had heard about the miracles that Jesus had performed in other people. Furthermore, the venue where Jesus taught was crowded with many people, but she didn't care. Observe the intensity of her desire to be healed in the following passage of Mark 5:27–29 (NKJV): "When she heard about Jesus, she came behind *Him* in the crowd and touched His garment. For she said, 'If only I may touch His clothes, I shall be made well.' Immediately the fountain of her blood was dried up, and she felt in *her* body that she was healed of the affliction." Notice that she had *faith* that if she could get close to Jesus, she would be healed. She had developed her faith by hearing about some of the testimonies that had taken place in the lives of others and knew that her disease was not an exception. She had a desire to be healed and had faith that she would be healed, but notice that she released her faith by acting on what she believed. She *said* to herself, "If only I may touch His clothes, I shall be made well," and then she reached out and touched Jesus's garment. Remember what I said earlier about God having an aura of healing power flowing from Him? Jesus was so saturated with God's anointing power (the Holy Spirit) that it seeped out from Him onto His clothing, so when the woman touched His clothing, she was healed.

Another example of healing taking place because of having faith in God is found in the book of Acts. In Acts 3, the apostle Peter was walking to the temple to pray when he encountered a man who had been lame from birth. The man asked Peter for a donation, but Peter replied, "Silver and gold I do not have, but what I do have I give you: In the name of Jesus Christ of Nazareth, rise up and walk" (Acts 3:6 NJKV). As we read further, Peter "took him by the right hand and lifted *him* up, and immediately his feet and ankle bones received strength. So he, leaping up, stood and walked and entered the temple with them—walking, leaping, and praising God" (Acts 3:7–8 NKJV). When Peter was questioned about how this miracle occurred, he credited it to having faith in the name of Jesus. In the sixteenth verse of this chapter, Peter made the following statement: "And His name, through faith in His name, has made this man strong, whom you see and know. Yes, the faith which *comes* through Him has given him this perfect soundness in the presence of you all." One way to develop your faith in God and in the name of Jesus is to believe that God loves you. You're more likely to approach your natural father for a request if you are convinced that he loves you. God loves you and has made the name of Jesus Christ available to you. If you'll ask Him for anything in Jesus's name, He will do it.

Your Healing Depends on You, Not on God

The timing of your healing is not up to God but is up to you. Don't think that you're waiting on God to heal you; He is looking for your faith, and the moment you're ready to believe and release your faith is the moment that you can be made whole. In Mark 9, a father brought to Jesus his son who had been tormented by an evil spirit, which caused him to have seizures and fall into fire and water. The father petitioned Jesus with the following statement: "But if You can do anything, have compassion on us and help us" (Mark 9:22 NKJV). Jesus immediately replied, "If *you* can believe, all things *are* possible to him who believes" (Mark 9:23 NKJV, emphasis added). You receive your healing from God by believing that Jesus can and will heal you. You release your faith by using the name of Jesus and believing in His name. Here's a sample prayer.

> Dear heavenly father, I come to You in Jesus's name for healing in my wrists. Your Word tells me in Mark 9:23 that if I can believe, all things are possible to me. I receive my healing now and thank You for it in Jesus's name. Amen.

Eliminating Healing Blockers

Although it is the perfect will of God in Christ Jesus to heal you, certain things may hinder you from receiving your healing from Him. Things that hinder your healing or healing blockers prevent God's healing power from flowing to you even though He has already made it available to everyone who asks for it. Some of these healing blockers include doubt, unbelief, fear, pride, bitterness, unforgiveness, strife, cheating, lying, hatred, sexual immorality, or any other form of sin. God doesn't desire to condemn you if any of these categories apply to you, but sin of any form will separate you from Him and all the wonderful things that He has in store for you. Don't be fearful. All you must do is repent and ask Him to forgive you, and He will be faithful to do it. For some individuals, it's a temper problem. For others, it's having multiple sexual partners. For most people, it's telling a little "white lie."

Another area that is often overlooked, but is vital, is that of unforgiveness. It's sometimes difficult to pinpoint exactly how it develops. It starts out as hurt feelings, and if it's not dealt with, it grows into resentment. Unforgiveness is extremely detrimental to your health and can increase the possibility of health problems. No matter how little or big the sin is, confess it before the Lord, ask Him to forgive you of it, and ask for His grace to stop doing it. In 1 John 1:9 (NJKV), the Bible says, "If we confess our sins, He is faithful and just to forgive us *our* sins and to cleanse us from all unrighteousness." When you confess your sins, you open the door for restoration between you and the Lord to take place. As you do so, you also create the environment in which the Lord can help you get rid of that area of struggle in your life. In unforgiveness, it's important to attempt to seek forgiveness if you were the one who offended someone. Forgiveness is not just for the other person's benefit; it's also for your benefit. If possible, reconcile with the other person who offended you or whom you offended. When you identify any area of sin in your life, confess it to the Lord and stop doing it. God's love for you is bigger than any personal struggles that you may have, and His grace will help you to overcome them if you will allow it. Decide today to get rid of your own healing blockers so that the healing that Jesus paid for on the cross may be available to you without anything hindering it.

Practical Application

The same way that you faithfully take your medications daily, do so with healing scriptures. Identify the verses that apply to the situation you're facing, and then follow the instructions of Proverbs 4:20–22 and Joshua 1:8. Keep healing scriptures before your eyes, read them out loud or listen to sermons, and spend enough time with them that they take root in your heart. Speak out loud those scriptures, meditate on them day and night, and act on what you believe God to heal you of. You act on what you believe by speaking words that are in line with what you believe. Trust God to have and by having corresponding action to your faith. For example, once you've prayed for your healing, don't walk around any longer saying, "I feel so sick today." Instead say, "The symptoms may still be present, but I believe I receive my healing in Jesus's name." If you had lain in bed because you felt so sick after you prayed, make yourself get up even if it's for a little while. You see, you must take steps to demonstrate your faith, even if you don't feel like it and especially when those symptoms persist. Whether your healing comes immediately or over a period, always know that Jesus is the faithful healer.

To help you get started, I will provide a list of healing scriptures in the next chapter. For now, continue taking your prescribed medications but add several "doses" of healing scriptures to your daily regimen. Meditate on those verses every day, preferably in the morning and evening. Allow the promises of God to take deep root inside your heart so that faith in God and faith in the name of Jesus can be developed. I do not recommend that you stop taking your medications until you first speak with your physician. Certain medications may have to be weaned off gradually to prevent serious, life-threatening effects. Also, keep a journal entry of your progress so that you're reminded of the improvements you've had so far, and don't become discouraged. In addition to meditating on healing scriptures, spend time daily praising and worshipping God. Read the book of Psalms, especially Psalms 91, 92, 103, and 144–150 for praise inspiration. There are certain matters of the heart that only the presence of God can effectively penetrate through and produce healing.

If you've experienced significant improvements in your health and wish to discontinue taking your medications, again I caution you to do so under a physician's supervision. The most important thing that I want to emphasize is putting your faith in God. Believe God that you are healed of every symptom and keep taking your medications until you are well enough to come off them. Believe the love that God has for you. The same God who strategically designed certain plants to minister health to you is the same being who wants to have a significant impact on your health crisis. He has made the Bible and the name of Jesus available to you. Take advantage of the opportunity that He has placed before you today. Before you head to the next chapter, here are some true stories that will encourage your faith in believing God for your healing.

Examples of Faith

One of the first examples that I will provide involves myself. As you can probably tell, I believe in practicing what I preach. One day, I was getting ready for bed and got under my blanket, ready to rest my head. I don't know if it was because of something I ate, but suddenly, I became so dizzy and didn't feel good. I had never experienced anything quite like this before. I usually sleep with my phone by my side, so I opened my Bible app and selected Isaiah 53:4–5 in the Amplified Bible Classic Edition, one of my go-to healing scriptures. I read the verses out loud and meditated on them. I went over them twice and believed them. Within minutes, the dizziness went away. I felt better and fell asleep. It was that easy.

Whether you are dealing with physical sickness or emotional distress, it makes no difference to the Lord. His ears are always open to the requests of His people. A few years ago, one of my staff shared with me that she had difficulty sleeping because she was afraid to sleep. As I inquired further, she mentioned that there was something in her home that had tried to choke her a few times (believe me, this is very real). Please listen carefully. It was not a family member who was doing this; something demonic was attacking her in her home, interrupting her sleep. I replied to her, "Say, 'In the name of Jesus, I command you to leave!'" She agreed to do so. A few weeks later when I saw the young girl again, I asked her how she was doing and whether her sleep patterns were different. She replied with a big smile, "I did what you said and am no longer afraid at night. I now have faith in the name of Jesus." In this circumstance, I gave her words to speak that were based on Scripture. She wasn't necessarily sure that it would work, but because I had recommended it, she did it and got her desired result.

This next example involves a relative of mine who had experienced a relapse of mental illness. For many years of her life, she would experience it on and off. Her illness was usually well controlled with medication, but whenever she was sick with a cold or flu for an extended period, the symptoms resurfaced. Whenever it occurred, it was always very devastating to our family. Several years ago, on a Sunday morning, I was on my way to church when I received a text message from one of my family members that this individual had relapsed. What made it even more serious was that she was requesting to be taken back to her country of origin that very day. As I am telling this story, it is difficult for me to remain composed because the event had such a tremendous impact on me. I began receiving text messages from other members of the family saying that they were heading to the individual's home to say good-bye before her sibling came to take her back to her country of origin. I don't know how I managed to sit through the entire church service, but I did. At one point, I cried out to the Lord and wept greatly. After church was over, my best friend, who had also attended the service, contacted me, and I shared with her what had happened. Together, we took communion, declaring the name of Jesus and the blood of Jesus over my relative. We stood on the promise of 1 Corinthians 11:26 and believed that the body of Jesus had been broken for this situation and His blood had been poured out so that my relative could be healed. We prayed the prayer of faith, and I traveled about two hours to visit her. By the time I had arrived, every symptom of relapse was completely gone. She was in her right mind, and we gathered together as a family to pray. When she visited her psychiatrist the next day, she received a good report. As you can guess, this individual is still in residing in her current home. In this example, my best friend and I based our prayer of agreement on the Word of God, and we exercised our faith by believing that we would receive our petition the moment we prayed.

This last example of faith is a little humorous but nevertheless a true event. Do you know that God has a sense of humor? As you read further, you will agree. I was at a restaurant with a close friend of many years, and she shared the following story with me. For a day or two, she had noticed that her cat wasn't bouncing around like it usually did and knew from previous experiences with the cat that it was feeling ill. She had been learning about how to believe God for healing based on the promises of Scripture, so she decided to test it on her cat. According to her, she laid her hands on her cat and spoke healing passages over it. Within a short period, the cat returned to its normal habits.

In these four examples, you notice a common theme. Based on the promises of the Word of God, healing of the body, emotions, and mind was attained when faith was applied and exercised. As stated before, God is not a respecter of persons. What He is looking for is your faith to believe that He can heal you. Whether you need healing for your loved ones, yourself, or even your pet, if you can believe, all things are possible. Now, you are prepared for the next chapter. As you read through the different categories of healing scriptures, identify the ones that apply to you and put them into practice today. Remember to read them out loud daily and trust God to do what He said He would do. Receive the healing that Jesus Christ has already made available to you.

Chapter 8: Healing Scriptures for Every Area of Life

Addictions (Drugs, Tobacco, Pornography, Drunkenness, Gluttony, and More)

1. For He satisfies the longing soul and fills the hungry soul with good. (Ps. 107:9 AMPC)
2. [The Lord] raises the poor out of the dust *and* lifts the needy from the ash heap *and* the dung hill, that He may seat them with princes, even with the princes of His people. (Ps. 113:7–8 AMPC)
3. For the law of the Spirit of life in Christ Jesus has made me free from the law of sin and death. (Rom. 8:2 NKJV)
4. Do you not know that your bodies are members of Christ?… Or do you not know that your body is the temple of the Holy Spirit *who is* in you, whom you have from God, and you are not your own? For you were bought at a price; therefore glorify God in your body and in your spirit, which are God's. (1 Cor. 6:15, 19–20 NKJV)

5. Who delivered us from so great a death, and does deliver us; in whom we trust that He will still deliver *us*. (2 Cor. 1:10 NKJV)

6. And He put all *things* under His feet, and gave Him *to be* head over all *things* to the church. (Eph. 1:21–22 NKJV)

7. He has delivered us from the power of darkness and conveyed *us* into the kingdom of the Son of His love. (Col. 1:13 NKJV)

8. And the Lord will deliver me from every evil work and preserve *me* for His heavenly kingdom. To Him *be* glory forever and ever. Amen! (2 Tim. 4:18 NKJV)

9. But we see Jesus, who was made a little lower than the angels, for the suffering of death crowned with glory and honor, that He, by the grace of God, might taste death for everyone…. That through death He might destroy him who had the power of death, that is, the devil, and release those who through fear of death were all their lifetime subject to bondage. (Heb. 2:9, 14–15 NKJV)

Aging/Old Age

1. Then the Lord said, My Spirit shall not forever dwell *and* strive with man, for he also is flesh; but his days shall yet be 120 years. (Gen. 6:3 AMPC)

2. Now as for you, you shall go to your fathers in peace; you shall be buried at a good old age. (Gen. 15:15 NKJV)

3. So you shall serve the Lord your God, and He will bless your bread and your water. And I will take sickness away from the midst of you…. I will fulfill the number of your days. (Exo. 23:25–26 NKJV)

4. Your sandals *shall be* iron and bronze; as your days, *so shall* your strength *be*. (Deut. 33:25 NKJV)
5. You shall come to the grave at a full age, as a sheaf of grain ripens in its season. (Job 5:26 NKJV)
6. With long life I will satisfy him, and show him My salvation. (Ps. 91:16 NKJV)
7. The righteous shall flourish like a palm tree, he shall grow like a cedar in Lebanon. Those who are planted in the house of the Lord shall flourish in the courts of our God. They shall still bear fruit in old age; they shall be fresh and flourishing. (Ps. 92:12–14 NKJV)
8. Hear, my son, and receive my sayings, and the years of your life will be many. (Prov. 4:10 NKJV)
9. Even the youths shall faint and be weary, and the young men shall utterly fall, but those who wait on the Lord shall renew *their* strength; they shall mount up with wings like eagles, they shall run and not be weary, they shall walk and not faint. (Isa. 40:30–31 NKJV)
10. Even to *your* old age, I *am* He, and *even* to gray hairs I will carry *you!* I have made, and I will bear; even I will carry, and will deliver *you*. (Isa. 46:4 NKJV)

Anxiety and Anxiety-Related Disorders (PTSD, OCD, Panic Disorder, and More)

1. I will not be afraid of ten thousands of people, who have set *themselves* against me all around. (Ps. 3:6 NKJV)
2. I have set the Lord continually before me; because He is at my right hand, I shall not be moved. (Ps. 16:8 AMPC)

3. Some trust in *and* boast of chariots and some of horses, but we will trust in *and* boast of the name of the Lord our God. (Ps. 20:7 AMPC)

4. Yes, though I walk through the [deep, sunless] valley of the shadow of death, I will fear *or* dread no evil, for You are with me; Your rod [to protect] and Your staff [to guide], they comfort me. (Ps. 23:4 AMPC)

5. Wait *and* hope for *and* expect the Lord; be brave *and* of good courage and let your heart be stout *and* enduring. Yes, wait for *and* hope for *and* expect the Lord. (Ps. 27:14 AMPC)

6. In the multitude of my [anxious] thoughts within me, Your comforts cheer *and* delight my soul! (Ps. 94:19 AMPC)

7. Great peace have they who love Your law; nothing shall offend them *or* make them stumble. (Ps. 119:165 AMPC)

8. Those who trust in, lean on, *and* confidently hope in the Lord are like Mount Zion, which cannot be moved but abides *and* stands fast forever. (Ps. 125 AMPC)

9. It is vain for you to rise up early, to take rest late, to eat the bread of [anxious] toil—for He gives [blessings] to His beloved in sleep. (Ps. 127:2 AMPC)

10. Humble yourselves therefore under the mighty hand of God, that he may exalt you in due time: casting all your care upon him; for He careth for you. (1 Peter 5:6–7 KJV)

Attention Difficulties (ADHD, ADD, Racing Thoughts, Difficulty Controlling Your Thoughts)

1. A calm *and* undisturbed mind *and* heart are the life *and* health of the body, but envy, jealousy, *and* wrath are like rottenness of the bones. (Prov. 14:30 AMPC)
2. You will keep him in perfect peace, whose mind is stayed on You, because he trusts in You. (Isa. 26:3 NKJV)
3. But this *is* the covenant that I will make with the house of Israel after those days, says the Lord: I will put My law in their minds, and write it on their hearts; and I will be their God, and they shall be My people. (Jer. 31:33 NKJV)
4. For those who live according to the flesh set their minds on the things of the flesh, but those *who live* according to the Spirit, the things of the Spirit. For to be carnally minded *is* death, but to be spiritually minded *is* life and peace. (Rom. 8:5–6 NLT)
5. For, "Who can know the Lord's thoughts? Who knows enough to teach him?" But we understand these things, for we have the mind of Christ. (1 Cor. 2:16 NLT)
6. Pay careful attention to your own work, for then you will get the satisfaction of a job well done, and you won't need to compare yourself to anyone else. (Gal. 6:4 NLT)
7. No, dear brothers and sisters, I have not achieved it, but I focus on this one thing: Forgetting the past and looking forward to what lies ahead, I press on to reach the end of the race and receive the heavenly prize for which God, through Christ Jesus, is calling us. (Phil. 3:13 NLT)

8. Finally, brethren, whatever things are true, whatever things are noble, whatever things are just, whatever things are pure, whatever things are lovely, whatever things are of good report, if there is any virtue and if there is anything praiseworthy—meditate on these things. (Phil. 4:8 NKJV)

9. If then you were raised with Christ, seek those things which are above, where Christ is, sitting at the right hand of God. Set your mind on things above, not on things on the earth. (Col. 3:1–2 NKJV)

10. For God did not give us a spirit of timidity (of cowardice, of craven and cringing and fawning fear), but [He has given us a spirit] of power and of love and of calm *and* well-balanced mind *and* discipline *and* self-control. (2 Tim. 1:7 AMPC)

Asthma, Bronchitis, COPD, Breathing Difficulties

1. When You send forth Your Spirit *and* give them breath, they are created, and You replenish the face of the ground. (Ps. 104:30 AMPC)

2. Thus says the Lord God to these bones: "Surely I will cause breath to enter into you, and you shall live." (Ezek. 37:5 NKJV)

3. I will put My Spirit in you, and you shall live, and I will place you in your own land. Then you shall know that I, the Lord, have spoken *it* and performed *it,* says the Lord. (Ezek. 37:14 NKJV)

4. For thus says the Lord to the house of Israel: "Seek Me and live." (Amos 5:4 NKJV)

5. And Jesus went about all Galilee, teaching in their synagogues, preaching the gospel of the kingdom,

> and healing all kinds of sickness and all kinds of disease among the people. (Matt. 4:23 NKJV)

6. But when Jesus knew *it,* He withdrew from there. And great multitudes followed Him, and He healed them all. (Matt. 12:15 NKJV)

7. It is the Spirit who gives life; the flesh profits nothing. The words that I speak to you are spirit, and *they* are life. (John 6:63 NKJV)

8. The thief does not come except to steal, and to kill, and to destroy. I have come that they may have life, and that they may have *it* more abundantly. (John 10:10 NKJV)

9. If you ask anything in My name, I will do *it.* (John 14:14 NKJV)

10. Jesus Christ *is* the same yesterday, today, and forever. (Heb. 13:8 NKJV)

Authority

(You have authority over sickness and disease in the name of Jesus Christ)

1. What is man that You are mindful of him, and the son of [earthborn] man that You care for him? Yet You have made him but a little lower than God [or heavenly beings], and You have crowned him with glory and honor. You made him to have dominion over the works of Your hands; You have put all things under his feet. (Ps. 8:6 AMPC)

2. "No weapon formed against you shall prosper, and every tongue which rises against you in judgment you shall condemn. This is the heritage of the servants of

the Lord, and their righteousness is from Me," says the Lord. (Isa. 54:17 NKJV)

3. And these signs will follow those who believe: In My name they will cast out demons; they will speak with new tongues; they will take up serpents; and if they drink anything deadly, it will by no means hurt them; they will lay hands on the sick, and they will recover. (Mark 16:17–18 NKJV)

4. And they were astonished at His teaching, for His word was with authority. (Luke 4:32 NKJV)

5. Then He [Jesus] called His twelve disciples together and gave them power and authority over all demons, and to cure diseases. He sent them to preach the kingdom of God and to heal the sick. (Luke 9:1–2 NKJV)

6. Behold, I give you the authority to trample on serpents and scorpions, and over all the power of the enemy, and nothing shall by any means hurt you. (Luke 10:19 NKJV)

7. But God, who is rich in mercy, because of His great love with which He loved us, even when we were dead in trespasses, made us alive together with Christ (by grace you have been saved), and raised us up together, and made us sit together in the heavenly places in Christ Jesus. (Eph. 2:4–7 NKJV)

Blood, Menstrual Disorders, Heart-Related Diseases

All diseases that affect the blood or the heart, which pumps blood, such as hypertension, bleeding disorders, blood clots, heart attacks, and more. This section also covers sepsis and organisms that infect the blood. Some of the Bible verses will deal with the cleansing of blood.

1. The poor shall eat and be satisfied; those who seek Him will praise the LORD. Let your heart live forever! (Ps. 22:26 NKJV)

2. O God, my heart is fixed (steadfast, in the confidence of faith); I will sing, yes, I will sing praises, even with my glory [all the faculties and powers of one created in Your image]! (Ps. 108:1 AMPC)

3. And when I passed by you and saw you struggling in your own blood, I said to you in your blood, "Live!" Yes, I said to you in your blood, "Live!" (Ezek. 16:6 NKJV)

4. Then I washed you in water; yes, I thoroughly washed off your blood, and I anointed you with oil. (Ezek. 16:9 NKJV)

5. Now a certain woman had a flow of blood for twelve years, and had suffered many things from many physicians. She had spent all that she had and was no better, but rather grew worse. When she heard about Jesus, she came behind *Him* in the crowd and touched His garment. For she said, "If only I may touch His clothes, I shall be made well." Immediately the fountain of her blood was dried up, and she felt in *her* body that she was healed of the affliction. (Mark 5:25–29 NKJV)

6. Now, Lord, look on their threats, and grant to Your servants that with all boldness they may speak Your word, by stretching out Your hand to heal, and that signs and wonders may be done through the name of Your holy Servant Jesus. (Acts 4:30 NKJV)

7. Because God's children are human beings—made of flesh and blood—the Son also became flesh and blood. For only as a human being could He die, and only by dying could He break the power of the devil, who had the power of death. Only in this way could He set free all who have lived their lives as slaves to the fear of dying. (Heb. 2:14–15 NLT)

8. And it came to pass, that the father of Publius lay sick of a fever and of a bloody flux: to whom Paul entered in, and prayed, and laid his hands on him, and healed him. So when this was done, others also, which had diseases in the island, came, and were healed. (Acts 28:8–9 KJV)

9. Christ also loved the church and gave Himself for her, that He might sanctify and cleanse her with the washing of water by the word. (Eph. 5:25–26 NKJV)

10. Beloved, I pray that you may prosper in all things and be in health, just as your soul prospers. (3 John 2 NKJV)

Bones, Bone-Related Diseases (Osteoporosis, Osteomyelitis, Osteomalacia, and More)

1. Have mercy on me, O Lord, for I *am* weak; O Lord, heal me, for my bones are troubled. (Ps. 6:2 NKJV)

2. Many *are* the afflictions of the righteous, but the LORD delivers him out of them all. He guards all his bones; not one of them is broken. (Ps. 34:19–20 NKJV)

3. All my bones shall say, Lord, who is like You, You Who deliver the poor *and* the afflicted from him who is too strong for him, yes, the poor and the needy from him who snatches away his goods? (Ps. 35:10 AMPC)

4. Do not be wise in your own eyes; Fear the Lord and depart from evil. It will be health to your flesh, and strength to your bones. (Prov. 3:8 NKJV)

5. The light of the eyes rejoices the heart, a*nd* a good report makes the bones healthy. (Prov. 15:30 NKJV)

6. Pleasant words *are like* a honeycomb, sweetness to the soul and health to the bones. (Prov. 16:24 NKJV)

7. "For I will restore health to you and heal you of your wounds," says the Lord, "because they called you an outcast *saying:* 'This *is* Zion; no one seeks her.'" (Jer. 30:17 NKJV)

8. He asked me, "Son of man, can these bones live?" I said, "Sovereign Lord, you alone know." Then He said to me, "Prophesy to these bones and say to them, 'Dry bones, hear the word of the Lord! This is what the Sovereign Lord says to these bones: I will make breath enter you, and you will come to life. I will attach tendons to you and make flesh come upon you and cover you with skin; I will put breath in you, and you will come to life. Then you will know that I am the Lord.'" So I prophesied as I was commanded. And as I was prophesying, there was a noise, a rattling sound, and the bones came together, bone to bone. (Ezek. 37:3–7 NIV)

9. And His [Jesus] name, through faith in His name, has made this man strong, whom you see and know. Yes, the faith which comes through Him has given him this perfect soundness in the presence of you all. (Acts 3:16 NKJV)

10. And Peter said to him, "Aeneas, Jesus the Christ heals you. Arise and make your bed." Then he arose immediately. (Acts 9:34 NKJV)

Crippled, Lame

1. The Lord opens the eyes of the blind, the Lord lifts up those who are bowed down, the Lord loves the [uncompromisingly] righteous (those upright in heart and in right standing with Him). (Ps. 146:8 AMPC)

2. Then the lame shall leap like a deer, and the tongue of the dumb sing. For waters shall burst forth in the wilderness, and streams in the desert. (Isa. 35:6 NKJV)

3. Then great multitudes came to Him, having with them the lame, blind, mute, maimed, and many others; and they laid them down at Jesus's feet, and He healed them. (Matt. 15:30 NKJV)

4. Then the blind and the lame came to Him in the temple, and He healed them. (Matt. 21:14 NKJV)

5. Jesus went into the synagogue again and noticed a man with a deformed hand.… Jesus said to the man with the deformed hand, "Come and stand in front of everyone." Then He said to the man, "Hold out your hand." So the man held out his hand, and it was restored! (Mark 3:1–5 NLT)

6. Then He [Jesus] told John's disciples, "Go back to John and tell him what you have seen and heard—the blind see, the lame walk, those with leprosy are cured, the deaf hear, the dead are raised to life, and the Good News is being preached to the poor." (Luke 7:22 NLT)

7. Crowds of sick people—blind, lame, or paralyzed—lay on the porches. One of the men lying there had been sick for thirty-eight years. When Jesus saw him and knew he had been ill for a long time … Jesus told him, "Stand up, pick up your mat, and walk!" Instantly, the

man was healed! He rolled up his sleeping mat and began walking! (John 5:3–9 NLT)

8. The lame man looked at them eagerly, expecting some money. But Peter said, "I don't have any silver or gold for you. But I'll give you what I have. In the name of Jesus Christ the Nazarene, get up and walk!" Then Peter took the lame man by the right hand and helped him up. And as he did, the man's feet and ankles were instantly healed and strengthened. (Acts 3:5–7 NLT)

9. Crowds listened intently to Philip because they were eager to hear his message and see the miraculous signs he did. Many evil spirits were cast out, screaming as they left their victims. And many who had been paralyzed or lame were healed. (Acts 8:6–7 NLT)

10. Therefore strengthen the hands which hang down, and the feeble knees, and make straight paths for your feet, so that what is lame may not be dislocated, but rather be healed. (Heb. 12:12–13 NKJV)

Communicable Diseases (Flu, Common Cold, and All Other Bacterial, Viral, Fungal, and Protozoal infections)

1. If you diligently heed the voice of the LORD your God and do what is right in His sight, give ear to His commandments and keep all His statutes, I will put none of the diseases on you which I have brought on the Egyptians. For I *am* the LORD who heals you. (Exo. 15:26 NKJV)

2. No evil shall befall you, nor shall any plague come near your dwelling. (Ps. 91:10 NKJV)

3. Who forgives [every one of] all your iniquities, Who heals [each one of] all your diseases. (Ps. 103:3 AMPC)

4. "For I will restore health to you, and I will heal your wounds," says the Lord, "because they have called you an outcast, saying, 'This is Zion, whom no one seeks after *and* for whom no one cares!'" (Jer. 30:17 AMPC)

5. Then Jesus put out *His* hand and touched him, saying, "I am willing; be cleansed." Immediately his leprosy was cleansed. (Matt. 8:3 NKJV)

6. That it might be fulfilled which was spoken by Isaiah the prophet, saying: "He Himself took our infirmities and bore our sicknesses." (Matt. 8:17 NKJV)

7. When Jesus heard *that,* He said to them, "Those who are well have no need of a physician, but those who are sick." (Matt. 9:12 NKJV)

8. And these signs will follow those who believe: In My name they will cast out demons; they will speak with new tongues; they will take up serpents; and if they drink anything deadly, it will by no means hurt them; they will lay hands on the sick, and they will recover. (Mark 16:17–18 NKJV)

9. Now God worked unusual miracles by the hands of Paul, so that even handkerchiefs or aprons were brought from his body to the sick, and the diseases left them and the evil spirits went out of them. (Acts 19:11–12 NKJV)

10. Christ also loved the church and gave Himself for her, that He might sanctify and cleanse her with the washing of water by the word. (Eph. 5:25–26 NKJV)

Deliverance from Troubled Situations

1. Salvation belongs to the Lord; May Your blessing be upon Your people. *Selah* [pause, and calmly think of that]! (Ps. 3:8 AMPC)

2. My voice You shall hear in the morning, O Lord; in the morning I will direct *it* to You, and I will look up. (Ps. 5:3 NKJV)

3. The Lord has heard my supplication; the Lord receives my prayer. (Ps. 6:9 AMPC)

4. When my enemies turn back, they shall fall and perish at Your presence. For You have maintained my right and my cause; You sat on the throne judging in righteousness. (Ps. 9:3–4 NKJV)

5. The Lord also will be a refuge for the oppressed, a refuge in times of trouble. (Ps. 9:9 NKJV) "For the oppression of the poor, for the sighing of the needy, now I will arise," says the LORD; "I will set him in the safety for which he yearns." (Ps. 12:5 NKJV)

6. I have set the Lord continually before me; because He is at my right hand, I shall not be moved. Therefore my heart is glad and my glory [my inner self] rejoices; my body too shall rest and confidently dwell in safety. (Ps. 16:8–9 AMPC)

7. Because he has set his love upon Me, therefore I will deliver him; I will set him on high, because he has known My name. He shall call upon Me, and I will answer him; I will be with him in trouble; I will deliver him and honor him. (Ps. 91:14–15 NKJV)

8. I will lift up my eyes to the hills—From whence comes my help? My help comes from the Lord, who made heaven and earth. (Ps. 121:1–2 NKJV) I wait for the Lord, my soul waits, and in His word I do hope. My soul waits for the Lord more than those who watch for the morning—yes, more than those who watch for the morning. (Ps. 130:5–6 NKJV)

Dementia, Memory Impairment, Difficulty Remembering Things

1. Sing praise to the Lord, you saints of His, And give thanks at the remembrance of His holy name. (Ps. 30:4 NKJV)
2. I call to remembrance my song in the night; I meditate within my heart, and my spirit makes diligent search. (Ps. 77:6 NKJV)
3. But then I recall all you have done, O Lord; I remember your wonderful deeds of long ago. (Ps. 77:11 NLT)
4. He has made His wonderful works to be remembered; the Lord is gracious, merciful, and full of loving compassion. (Ps. 111:4 AMPC)
5. The memory of the righteous *is* blessed, But the name of the wicked will rot. (Prov. 10:7 NKJV)
6. As for you, O king, thoughts came *to* your *mind while* on your bed, *about* what would come to pass after this; and He who reveals secrets has made known to you what will be. (Dan. 2:29 NKJV)
7. But the Helper, the Holy Spirit, whom the Father will send in My name, He will teach you all things, and bring to your remembrance all things that I said to you. (John 14:26 NKJV)
8. 8. No longer do I call you servants, for a servant does not know what his master is doing; but I have called you friends, for all things that I heard from My Father I have made known to you. (John 15:15 NKJV)
9. You have made known to me the ways of life; You will make me full of joy in Your presence. (Acts 2:28 NKJV)
10. But you have an anointing from the Holy One, and you know all things. (1 John 2:20 NKJV)

Depression or Depressed State due to Sadness, Sorrow, Broken Heart, and More

1. Depart from me, all you workers of iniquity, for the Lord has heard the voice of my weeping. The Lord has heard my supplication; the Lord receives my prayer. (Ps. 6:8–9 AMPC)
2. I will extol You, O Lord, for You have lifted me up and have not let my foes rejoice over me. O Lord my God, I cried to You and You have healed me. (Ps. 30:1–2 AMPC)
3. For His anger is but for a moment, but His favor is for a lifetime *or* in His favor is life. Weeping may endure for a night, but joy comes in the morning. (Ps. 30:5 AMPC)
4. You have turned for me my mourning into dancing; You have put off my sackcloth and clothed me with gladness, to the end that *my* glory may sing praise to You and not be silent. O Lord my God, I will give thanks to You forever. (Ps. 30:11–12 NKJV)
5. *The righteous* cry out, and the Lord hears, and delivers them out of all their troubles. The Lord *is* near to those who have a broken heart, and saves such as have a contrite spirit. (Ps. 34:17–18 NKJV)
6. Why are you cast down, O my soul? And *why* are you disquieted within me? Hope in God, for I shall yet praise Him *for* the help of His countenance. (Ps. 42:5 NKJV) Father to the fatherless, defender of widows— this is God, whose dwelling is holy. (Ps. 68:5 NLT)
7. For You have delivered my soul from death, my eyes from tears, a*nd* my feet from falling. (Ps. 116:8 NKJV)
8. He heals the brokenhearted and binds up their wounds. (Ps. 147:3 NKJV)

9. He will wipe every tear from their eyes, and there will be no more death or sorrow or crying or pain. All these things are gone forever. (Rev. 21:4 NLT)

Diabetes, Prediabetes

1. And God said, "See, I have given you every herb *that* yields seed which *is* on the face of all the earth, and every tree whose fruit yields seed; to you it shall be for food." (Gen. 1:29 NKJV)
2. When you have eaten and are full, then you shall bless the Lord your God for all the good land which He has given you. (Deut. 8:10 AMPC)
3. I call heaven and earth to witness this day against you that I have set before you life and death, the blessings and the curses; therefore choose life, that you and your descendants may live. (Deut. 30:19 AMPC)
4. Bless the Lord, O my soul, and forget not all His benefits: Who forgives all your iniquities, Who heals all your diseases. (Ps. 103:2–3 NKJV)
5. If you will only obey me, you will have plenty to eat. (Isa. 1:19 AMPC)
6. Say to the righteous that it shall be well with them, for they shall eat the fruit of their deeds. (Isa. 3:10 AMPC)
7. By the time this child is old enough to choose what is right and reject what is wrong, he will be eating yogurt and honey. (Isa. 7:15 NLT)
8. Why spend your money on food that does not give you strength? Why pay for food that does you no good? Listen to me, and you will eat what is good. You will enjoy the finest food. (Isa. 55:2 NLT)
9. Call to Me and I will answer you and show you great and mighty things, fenced in *and* hidden, which you

do not know (do not distinguish and recognize, have knowledge of and understand). (Jer. 33:3 AMPC)

9. But as for you, take wheat, barley, beans, lentils, millet, and spelt, and put them into one vessel and make them into bread for yourself. You shall eat it according to the number of the days that you lie on your side, three hundred and ninety days. (Ezek. 4:9 AMPC)

Eye Disorders (Glaucoma, Cataract, Blindness, Macular Degeneration, Diabetic Retinopathy)

1. Open my eyes to see the wonderful truths in your instructions. (Ps. 119:18 NLT)
2. The LORD opens the eyes of the blind. The LORD lifts up those who are weighed down. The LORD loves the godly. (Ps. 146:8 NLT)
3. Look straight ahead, and fix your eyes on what lies before you. (Prov. 4:25 NLT)
4. Ears to hear and eyes to see—both are gifts from the LORD. (Prov. 20:12 NLT)
5. In that day the deaf will hear words read from a book, and the blind will see through the gloom and darkness. (Isa. 29:18 NLT)
6. You will open the eyes of the blind. You will free the captives from prison, releasing those who sit in dark dungeons. (Isa. 42:7 NLT)
7. They went right into the house where he was staying, and Jesus asked them, "Do you believe I can make you see?" "Yes, Lord," they told him, "we do." Then he touched their eyes and said, "Because of your faith, it will happen." Then their eyes were opened, and they could see! (Matt. 9:28–30 NLT)

8. Jesus felt sorry for them and touched their eyes. Instantly they could see! Then they followed him. (Matt. 20:34 NLT)

9. Then Jesus placed his hands on the man's eyes again, and his eyes were opened. His sight was completely restored, and he could see everything clearly. (Mark 8:25 NLT)

10. The Spirit of the Lord *is* upon Me, because He has anointed Me to preach the gospel to *the* poor; he has sent Me to heal the brokenhearted, to proclaim liberty to *the* captives and recovery of sight to *the* blind. (Luke 4:18 NKJV)

Falls/Slipping

1. If I say, "My foot slips," Your mercy, O Lord, will hold me up. (Ps. 94:18 NKJV)

2. For He shall give His angels charge over you, to keep you in all your ways. In *their* hands they shall bear you up, lest you dash your foot against a stone. (Ps. 91:11–12 NKJV)

3. Return to your rest, O my soul, for the Lord has dealt bountifully with you. For You have delivered my soul from death, my eyes from tears, a*nd* my feet from falling. (Ps. 116:7–8 NKJV)

4. You pushed me violently, that I might fall, but the Lord helped me. (Ps. 118:13 NKJV)

5. Seven times a day I praise You, because of Your righteous judgments. Great peace have those who love Your law, and nothing causes them to stumble. (Ps. 119:164–165 NKJV)

6. My help comes from the Lord, Who made heaven and earth. He will not allow your foot to slip *or* to be moved; He Who keeps you will not slumber. (Ps. 121:2–3 AMPC)

Favor

1. For You, O Lord, will bless the righteous; with favor You will surround him as *with* a shield. (Ps. 5:12 NKJV)
2. For His anger *is but for* a moment, his favor *is for* life; weeping may endure for a night, but joy *comes* in the morning. (Ps. 30:5 NKJV)
3. Lord, by Your favor You have made my mountain stand strong; you hid Your face, *and* I was troubled. (Ps. 30:7 NKJV)
4. Blessed be the Lord! For He has shown me His marvelous loving favor when I was beset as in a besieged city. (Ps. 31:21 AMPC)
5. By this I know that You favor *and* delight in me, because my enemy does not triumph over me. (Ps. 41:11 AMPC)
6. Remember me, O LORD, with the favor *You have toward* Your people. Oh, visit me with Your salvation. (Ps. 106:4 NKJV)

Fear, Worry, Stress, Concerns

1. I will give peace in the land, and you shall lie down, and none will make *you* afraid; I will rid the land of evil beasts, and the sword will not go through your land. (Lev. 26:6 NKJV)
2. Be strong and of good courage, do not fear nor be afraid of them; for the LORD your God, He *is* the One who goes with you. He will not leave you nor forsake you. (Deut. 31:6 AMPC)

3. Commit your way to the Lord [roll and repose each care of your load on Him]; trust (lean on, rely on, and be confident) also in Him and He will bring it to pass. (Ps. 37:5 AMPC)

4. Be still *and* rest in the Lord; wait for Him *and* patiently lean yourself upon Him; fret not yourself because of him who prospers in his way, because of the man who brings wicked devices to pass. (Ps. 37:7 AMPC)

5. God is our refuge and strength, always ready to help in times of trouble. So we will not fear when earthquakes come and the mountains crumble into the sea. (Ps. 46:1–2 NLT)

6. Whenever I am afraid, I will trust in You. (Ps. 56:3 NKJV)

7. In God (I will praise His word), in God I have put my trust; I will not fear. What can flesh do to me? (Ps. 56:4 NKJV)

8. Trust in the Lord with all your heart, and lean not on your own understanding; in all your ways acknowledge Him, and He shall direct your paths. (Prov. 3:5–6 NKJV)

9. For I, the Lord your God, will hold your right hand, saying to you, "Fear not, I will help you." (Isa. 41:13 NKJV)

10. Therefore do not worry, saying, "What shall we eat?" or "What shall we drink?" or "What shall we wear?" For after all these things the Gentiles seek. For your heavenly Father knows that you need all these things. But seek first the kingdom of God and His righteousness, and all these things shall be added to you. (Matt. 6:31–33 NKJV)

11. So we may boldly say: "The Lord *is* my helper; I will not fear. What can man do to me?" (Heb. 13:6 NKJV)

Guilt

1. For I will acquit them of the guilt of bloodshed, whom I had not acquitted; For the Lord dwells in Zion. (Joel 3:21 NKJV)
2. But if you had known what *this* means, "I desire mercy and not sacrifice," you would not have condemned the guiltless. (Matt. 12:7 NKJV)
3. Therefore we were buried with Him through baptism into death, that just as Christ was raised from the dead by the glory of the Father, even so we also should walk in newness of life. (Rom. 6:4 NKJV)
4. Therefore, if anyone *is* in Christ, *he is* a new creation; old things have passed away; behold, all things have become new. (2 Cor. 5:17 NKJV)
5. And you, being dead in your trespasses and the uncircumcision of your flesh, He has made alive together with Him, having forgiven you all trespasses, having wiped out the handwriting of requirements that was against us, which was contrary to us. And He has taken it out of the way, having nailed it to the cross. (Col. 2:13–14 NKJV)
6. For Christ has not entered the holy places made with hands, *which are* copies of the true, but into heaven itself, now to appear in the presence of God for us; not that He should offer Himself often, as the high priest enters the Most Holy Place every year with blood of another—He then would have had to suffer often since the foundation of the world; but now, once at the end of the ages, He has appeared to put away sin by the sacrifice of Himself. (Heb. 9:24–26 NKJV)

7. Therefore, brethren, having boldness to enter the Holiest by the blood of Jesus, by a new and living way which He consecrated for us, through the veil, that is, His flesh, and *having* a High Priest over the house of God, let us draw near with a true heart in full assurance of faith, having our hearts sprinkled from an evil conscience and our bodies washed with pure water. (Heb. 10:19–22 NKJV)

8. If we confess our sins, He is faithful and just to forgive us *our* sins and to cleanse us from all unrighteousness. (1 John 1:9 NKJV)

Hearing Impairment

1. Ears to hear and eyes to see—both are gifts from the Lord. (Prov. 20:12 NLT) In that day the deaf will hear words read from a book, and the blind will see through the gloom and darkness. (Isa. 29:18 NLT) And when he comes, he will open the eyes of the blind and unplug the ears of the deaf. (Isa. 35:5 NLT)

2. Jesus told them, "Go back to John and tell him what you have heard and seen—the blind see, the lame walk, those with leprosy are cured, the deaf hear, the dead are raised to life, and the Good News is being preached to the poor." (Matt. 11:4–5 NLT) 5. Anyone with ears to hear should listen and understand! (Matt. 11:15 NLT)

3. A deaf man with a speech impediment was brought to him, and the people begged Jesus to lay his hands on the man to heal him. Jesus led him away from the crowd so they could be alone. He put his fingers into the man's ears. Then, spitting on his own fingers, he touched the man's tongue. Looking up to heaven,

he sighed and said, *"Ephphatha,"* which means, "Be opened!" Instantly the man could hear perfectly, and his tongue was freed so he could speak plainly! (Mark 7:32–35 NLT)

4. And they were astonished beyond measure, saying, "He has done all things well. He makes both the deaf to hear and the mute to speak." (Mark 7:37 NKJV)

5. When Jesus saw that the crowd of onlookers was growing, he rebuked the evil spirit. "Listen, you spirit that makes this boy unable to hear and speak," he said. "I command you to come out of this child and never enter him again!" Then the spirit screamed and threw the boy into another violent convulsion and left him. (Mark 9:25–26 NLT)

6. Then He told John's disciples, "Go back to John and tell him what you have seen and heard—the blind see, the lame walk, those with leprosy are cured, the deaf hear, the dead are raised to life, and the Good News is being preached to the poor." (Luke 7:22 NLT)

7. As His divine power has given to us all things that *pertain* to life and godliness, through the knowledge of Him who called us by glory and virtue. (2 Pet. 1:3 NKJV)

Infertility, Barrenness, Difficulty Conceiving

1. And the Lord asked Abraham, Why did Sarah laugh, saying, "Shall I really bear a child when I am so old?" Is anything too hard *or* too wonderful for the Lord? At the appointed time, when the season [for her delivery] comes around, I will return to you and Sarah shall have borne a son. (Gen. 18:13–14 AMPC)

2. None shall lose her young by miscarriage or be barren in your land; I will fulfill the number of your days. (Exo. 23:26 AMPC)

3. You shall be blessed above all peoples; there shall not be male or female barren among you, or among your cattle. (Deut. 7:14 AMPC)

4. And the Angel of the Lord appeared to the woman and said to her, "Behold, you are barren and have no children, but you shall become pregnant and bear a son." (Judges 13:3 AMPC)

5. Those who were full have hired themselves out for bread, but those who were hungry have ceased to hunger. The barren has borne seven, but she who has many children languishes *and* is forlorn. (1 Sam. 2:5 AMPC)

6. Elisha said, "At this season when the time comes round, you shall embrace a son." She said, "No, my lord, you man of God, do not lie to your handmaid." But the woman conceived and bore a son at that season the following year, as Elisha had said to her. (2 Kings 4:16–17 AMPC)

7. He gives the childless woman a family, making her a happy mother. (Ps. 113:9 NLT)

8. Behold, children are a heritage from the Lord, the fruit of the womb a reward. (Ps. 127:3 AMPC)

9. Your wife shall be like a fruitful vine in the innermost parts of your house; your children shall be like olive plants round about your table. (Ps. 128:3 AMPC)

10. And listen! Your relative Elizabeth in her old age has also conceived a son, and this is now the sixth month with her who was called barren. For with God nothing is ever impossible *and* no word from God shall

be without power *or* impossible of fulfillment. (Luke 1:36–37 AMPC)

Joy

1. You have put gladness in my heart, more than in the season that their grain and wine increased. (Ps. 4:7 NKJV)
2. You will show me the path of life; in Your presence is fullness of joy, at Your right hand there are pleasures forevermore. (Ps. 16:11 AMPC)
3. For His anger *is but for* a moment, His favor *is for* life; Weeping may endure for a night, but joy *comes* in the morning. (Ps. 30:5 NKJV)
4. He brought out His people with joy, His chosen ones with gladness. (Ps. 105:43 NKJV)
5. Then he said to them, "Go your way, eat the fat, drink the sweet, and send portions to those for whom nothing is prepared; for *this* day *is* holy to our Lord. Do not sorrow, for the joy of the Lord is your strength." (Neh. 8:10 NKJV)
6. Therefore with joy you will draw water from the wells of salvation. (Isa. 12:3 NKJV)
7. The Spirit of the Lord God *is* upon Me, because the Lord has anointed Me.… To console those who mourn in Zion, to give them beauty for ashes, the oil of joy for mourning, the garment of praise for the spirit of heaviness. (Isa. 61:1, 3 NKJV)
8. Instead of your shame *you shall have* double *honor,* and *instead of* confusion they shall rejoice in their portion. Therefore in their land they shall possess double; everlasting joy shall be theirs. (Isa. 61:7 NKJV)

9. These things I have spoken to you, that My joy may remain in you, and *that* your joy may be full. (John 15:11 NKJV)

10. Most assuredly, I say to you that you will weep and lament, but the world will rejoice; and you will be sorrowful, but your sorrow will be turned into joy. (John 16:20 NKJV)

Laughter

1. And Sarah said, "God has made me laugh, *and* all who hear will laugh with me." (Gen. 21:6 NKJV)

2. He will yet fill your mouth with laughing, and your lips with rejoicing. Those who hate you will be clothed with shame, and the dwelling place of the wicked will come to nothing. (Job 8:21–22 NKJV)

3. You have put gladness in my heart, more than in the season that their grain and wine increased. (Ps. 4:7 NKJV)

4. When the Lord brought back the captivity of Zion, we were like those who dream. Then our mouth was filled with laughter, and our tongue with singing. Then they said among the nations, "The Lord has done great things for them." (Ps. 126:1–2 NKJV)

5. A merry heart makes a cheerful countenance, but by sorrow of the heart the spirit is broken. (Prov. 15:13 NKJV)

6. For the despondent, every day brings trouble; for the happy heart, life is a continual feast. (Prov. 15:15 NLT)

7. A happy heart is good medicine *and* a cheerful mind works healing, but a broken spirit dries up the bones. (Prov. 17:22 AMPC)

8. "For I will restore health to you and heal you of your wounds," says the LORD.... Then out of them shall proceed thanksgiving and the voice of those who make merry; I will multiply them, and they shall not diminish; I will also glorify them, and they shall not be small. (Jer. 30:17, 19 NKJV)

9. Blessed *are you* who hunger now, for you shall be filled. Blessed *are you* who weep now, for you shall laugh. (Luke 6:21 NKJV)

Pain (All Conditions Associated with Pain, Swelling, or Inflammation), Emotional Pain

1. Your garments did not wear out on you, nor did your foot swell these forty years. (Deut. 8:4 NKJV)

2. My heart is severely pained within me, and the terrors of death have fallen upon me. Evening and morning and at noon I will pray, and cry aloud, and He shall hear my voice. He has redeemed my soul in peace from the battle that was against me, for there were many against me. (Ps. 55:4; 17–18 NKJV)

3. I love the LORD, because He has heard my voice and my supplications. Because He has inclined His ear to me, therefore I will call upon Him as long as I live. (Ps. 116:1–2 NKJV)

4. Return to your rest, O my soul, for the LORD has dealt bountifully with you. For You have delivered my soul from death, my eyes from tears, and my feet from falling. (Ps. 116:7–8 NKJV)

5. A peaceful heart leads to a healthy body; jealousy is like cancer in the bones. (Prov. 14:30 NLT)

6. For I consider that the sufferings of this present time are not worthy to be compared with the glory which shall be revealed in us. (Rom. 8:18 NKJV)
7. For the word of God is living and powerful, and sharper than any two-edged sword, piercing even to the division of soul and spirit, and of joints and marrow, and is a discerner of the thoughts and intents of the heart. (Heb. 4:12 NKJV)
8. Therefore strengthen the hands which hang down, and the feeble knees, and make straight paths for your feet, so that what is lame may not be dislocated, but rather be healed. (Heb. 12:12–13 NKJV)
9. Beloved, I pray that you may prosper in all things and be in health, just as your soul prospers. (3 John 2 NKJV)
10. And God will wipe away every tear from their eyes; there shall be no more death, nor sorrow, nor crying. There shall be no more pain, for the former things have passed away. (Rev. 21:4 NKJV)

Protection

1. Do not be afraid, Abram. I *am* your shield, your exceedingly great reward. (Gen. 15:1 NKJV)
2. *As for* God, His way *is* perfect; The word of the Lord *is* proven; He *is* a shield to all who trust in Him. (2 Sam. 22:31 NKJV)
3. The Lord is my rock and my fortress and my deliverer; My God, my strength, in whom I will trust; My shield and the horn of my salvation, my stronghold. (Ps. 18:2 NKJV)
4. The Lord *is* my strength and my shield; my heart trusted in Him, and I am helped; Therefore my heart

greatly rejoices, and with my song I will praise Him. (Ps. 28:7 NKJV)

5. For the Lord God *is* a sun and shield; The Lord will give grace and glory; No good *thing* will He withhold from those who walk uprightly. (Ps. 84:11 NKJV)

6. Surely He shall deliver you from the snare of the fowler and from the perilous pestilence. (Ps. 91:3 NKJV)

7. Behold, He who keeps Israel shall neither slumber nor sleep. The Lord *is* your keeper. The Lord *is* your shade at your right hand. The sun shall not strike you by day, nor the moon by night. (Ps. 121:4–6 AMPC)

8. Blessed *be* the LORD my Rock, Who trains my hands for war, *and* my fingers for battle—my lovingkindness and my fortress, my high tower and my deliverer, my shield and *the One* in whom I take refuge, Who subdues my people under me. (Ps. 144:1–2 NKJV)

9. Finally, my brethren, be strong in the Lord and in the power of His might. Put on the whole armor of God, that you may be able to stand against the wiles of the devil.… Therefore take up the whole armor of God, that you may be able to withstand in the evil day, and having done all, to stand. (Eph. 6:10–11, 13 NKJV)

Provision (Food, Clothing, Finances, Desires)

1. The Lord *is* my shepherd; I shall not want. (Ps. 23:1 NKJV)

2. Behold, the eye of the Lord *is* on those who fear Him, on those who hope in His mercy, to deliver their soul from death, and to keep them alive in famine. (Ps. 33:18–19 NKJV)

3. Oh, fear the LORD, you His saints! *There is* no want to those who fear Him. The young lions lack and suffer

hunger; but those who seek the Lord shall not lack any good *thing*. (Ps. 34:9–10 NKJV)

4. Your righteousness is like the mighty mountains, your justice like the ocean depths. You care for people and animals alike, O Lord. (Ps. 36:6 NLT)

5. They relish *and* feast on the abundance of Your house; and You cause them to drink of the stream of Your pleasures. (Ps. 36:8 AMPC)

6. Delight yourself also in the Lord, and He will give you the desires *and* secret petitions of your heart. (Ps. 37:4 AMPC)

7. I have been young and now am old, yet have I not seen the [uncompromisingly] righteous forsaken or their seed begging bread. All day long they are merciful *and* deal graciously; they lend, and their offspring are blessed. (Ps. 37:25–26 AMPC)

8. He has given food *and* provision to those who reverently *and* worshipfully fear Him; He will remember His covenant forever *and* imprint it [on His mind]. (Ps. 111:5 AMPC)

9. May the Lord give you increase more and more, you and your children. (Ps. 115:14 AMPC)

10. But seek first the kingdom of God and His righteousness, and all these things shall be added to you. (Matt. 6:33 NKJV)

Sleep Disturbances, Difficulty Sleeping

1. I will both lie down in peace, and sleep; for You alone, O Lord, make me dwell in safety. (Ps. 4:8 NKJV)

2. *It is* vain for you to rise up early, to sit up late, to eat the bread of sorrows; *For* so He gives His beloved sleep. (Ps. 127:2 NKJV)

3. When you lie down, you will not be afraid; yes, you will lie down and your sleep will be sweet. (Prov. 3:24 NKJV)

4. The sleep of a laboring man *is* sweet, whether he eats little or much. (Ecc. 5:12 NKJV)

5. After this I awoke and looked around, and my sleep was sweet to me. (Jer. 31:26 NKJV)

6. I will make a covenant of peace with them, and cause wild beasts to cease from the land; and they will dwell safely in the wilderness and sleep in the woods. (Ezek. 34:25 NKJV)

Speech Problems, Saying the Wrong Things

1. 1. Then Moses said to the Lord, "O my Lord, I *am* not eloquent, neither before nor since You have spoken to Your servant; but I *am* slow of speech and slow of tongue." So the Lord said to him, "Who has made man's mouth? Or who makes the mute, the deaf, the seeing, or the blind? *Have* not I, the Lord? Now therefore, go, and I will be with your mouth and teach you what you shall say." (Exo. 4:10–12 NKJV)

2. The Spirit of the Lord speaks through me; his words are upon my tongue. (2 Sam. 23:2 NLT)

3. My lips will speak no evil, and my tongue will speak no lies. (Job 27:4 NLT)

4. For my words are wise, and my thoughts are filled with insight. (Ps. 49:3 NLT)

5. Those who control their tongue will have a long life; opening your mouth can ruin everything. (Prov. 13:3 NLT)

6. A gentle answer deflects anger, but harsh words make tempers flare. The tongue of the wise makes

knowledge appealing, but the mouth of a fool belches out foolishness. (Prov. 15:1–2 NLT)

7. Death and life *are* in the power of the tongue, and those who love it will eat its fruit. (Prov. 18:21 NKJV)

8. Then the lame shall leap like a deer, and the tongue of the dumb sing. For waters shall burst forth in the wilderness, and streams in the desert. (Isa. 35:6 NKJV)

9. A vast crowd brought to Him people who were lame, blind, crippled, those who couldn't speak, and many others. They laid them before Jesus, and he healed them all. (Matt. 15:30 NLT)

Tumors, Growths, Cancer-Related Effects, All Chronic and Terminal Illnesses

1. The Lord will sustain, refresh, *and* strengthen him on his bed of languishing; all his bed You [O Lord] will turn, change, *and* transform in his illness. (Ps. 41:3 AMPC)

2. However, the hair of his head began to grow again after it had been shaven. (Judges 16:22 NKJV)

3. God is to us a God of deliverances *and* salvation; and to God the Lord belongs escape from death [setting us free]. (Ps. 68:20 AMPC)

4. O you who love the Lord, hate evil; He preserves the lives of His saints (the children of God), He delivers them out of the hand of the wicked. (Ps. 97:10 AMPC)

5. He sends forth His word and heals them and rescues them from the pit *and* destruction. (Ps. 107:20 AMPC)

6. For You have delivered my life from death, my eyes from tears, and my feet from stumbling *and* falling. I will walk before the Lord in the land of the living. (Ps. 116:8–9 AMPC)

7. I shall not die but live, and shall declare the works *and* recount the illustrious acts of the Lord. (Ps. 118:17 AMPC)
8. This is my comfort *and* consolation in my affliction: that Your word has revived me *and* given me life. (Ps. 119:50 AMPC)
9. I will never forget Your precepts, for by them You have given me life. (Ps. 119:93 NKJV)
10. When you pass through the waters, I *will be* with you; and through the rivers, they shall not overflow you. When you walk through the fire, you shall not be burned, nor shall the flame scorch you. (Isa. 43:2 NKJV)
11. Behold, I *am* the Lord, the God of all flesh. Is there anything too hard for Me? (Jer. 32:27 NKJV)

Weakness (Associated with Fatigue, Frequent Falls, Strokes, Paralysis, and More)

1. Then he said to them, "Go your way, eat the fat, drink the sweet, and send portions to those for whom nothing is prepared; for *this* day *is* holy to our Lord. Do not sorrow, for the joy of the Lord is your strength." (Neh. 8:10 NKJV)
2. The Lord will strengthen him on his bed of illness; You will sustain him on his sickbed. (Ps. 41:3 NKJV)
3. The Lord *is* my strength and song, and He has become my salvation. (Ps. 118:14 NKJV)
4. He gives power to the weak, and to *those who have* no might He increases strength. (Isa. 40:29 NKJV)
5. But those who wait on the Lord, shall renew *their* strength; they shall mount up with wings like eagles, they shall run and not be weary, they shall walk and not faint. (Isa. 40:31 NKJV)

6. Fear not, for I *am* with you; be not dismayed, for I *am* your God. I will strengthen you, yes, I will help you, I will uphold you with My righteous right hand. (Isa. 41:10 NKJV)

7. I will search for My lost ones who strayed away, and I will bring them safely home again. I will bandage the injured and strengthen the weak. (Ezek. 34:16 NLT)

8. Beat your plowshares into swords and your pruning hooks into spears; let the weak say, "I *am* strong." (Joel 3:10 NKJV)

9. Yet I will rejoice in the Lᴏʀᴅ, I will joy in the God of my salvation. The Lᴏʀᴅ God is my strength; He will make my feet like deer's *feet,* and He will make me walk on my high hills. (Hab. 3:18–19 NKJV)

10. And His name, through faith in His name, has made this man strong, whom you see and know. Yes, the faith which *comes* through Him has given him this perfect soundness in the presence of you all. (Acts 3:16 NKJV)

Wisdom

1. The fear of the Lord *is* the beginning of wisdom; a good understanding have all those who do *His command-ments.* His praise endures forever. (Ps. 11:10 NKJV)

2. For with You *is* the fountain of life; in Your light we see light. (Ps. 36:9 NKJV)

3. The steps of a *good* man are ordered by the Lord, and He delights in his way. Though he fall, he shall not be utterly cast down; for the Lord upholds *him with* His hand. (Ps. 37:23–24 NKJV

4. The mouth of the righteous speaks wisdom, and his tongue talks of justice. The law of his God *is* in his heart; none of his steps shall slide. (Ps. 37:30–31 NKJV)

5. Behold, You desire truth in the inner being; make me therefore to know wisdom in my inmost heart. (Ps. 51:6 AMPC)

6. You will guide me with Your counsel, and afterward receive me to honor *and* glory. (Ps. 73:24 AMPC)

7. Teach me Your way, O Lord, that I may walk *and* live in Your truth; direct *and* unite my heart [solely, reverently] to fear *and* honor Your name. (Ps. 86:11 AMPC)

8. You, through Your commandments, make me wiser than my enemies; for they *are* ever with me. I have more understanding than all my teachers, for Your testimonies *are* my meditation. I understand more than the ancients, because I keep Your precepts. (Ps. 119:98–100 NKJV)

9. The entrance of Your words gives light; it gives understanding to the simple.…Direct my steps by Your word, and let no iniquity have dominion over me. (Psalm 119:130, 133 NKJV)

10. If any of you lacks wisdom, let him ask of God, who gives to all liberally and without reproach, and it will be given to him. (James 1:5 NKJV)

Notes

Chapter 1

1   Steven D. Ehrlich, "Herbal Medicine," University of Maryland Medical Center, last modified November 6, 2015, accessed July 1, 2017, http://www.umm.edu/health/medical/altmed/treatment/herbal-medicine.

2   "History of Medicine," Stonybrook University, accessed July 1, 2017, http://www.stonybrook.edu/bioethics/historyofmedicine.shtml.

3   *Encyclopædia Britannica*, s.v. "History of medicine," last modified June 14, 2017, accessed July 29, 2017, https://www.britannica.com/topic/history-of-medicine/Traditional-medicine-and-surgery-in-Asia.

4   The MNT Editorial Team, "What Is Ancient Egyptian Medicine?" *Healthline Media*, last modified January 5, 2016, accessed July 1, 2017, http://www.medicalnewstoday.com/info/medicine/ancient-egyptian-medicine.php.

5   The MNT Editorial Team, "What Is Ancient Greek Medicine?" *Healthline Media*, last modified January 5, 2016, accessed July 1, 2017, http://www.medicalnewstoday.com/info/medicine/ancient-greek-medicine.php.

6   The MNT Editorial Team, "What Is Ancient Roman Medicine?" *Healthline Media*, last modified January 5, 2016, accessed July 1, 2017, http://www.medicalnewstoday.com/info/medicine/ancient-roman-medicine.php.

7   The MNT Editorial Team, "What is Ancient Roman Medicine?"

8   The MNT Editorial Team, "What is Ancient Roman Medicine?"

9   The MNT Editorial Team, "What Is European Medieval and Renaissance Medicine?" *Healthline Media*, last modified January 5, 2016, accessed July 1, 2017, http://www.medicalnewstoday.com/info/medicine/medieval-and-renaissance-medicine.php.

10   The MNT Editorial Team, "What Is European Medieval and Renaissance Medicine?"

11   The MNT Editorial Team, "What Is European Medieval and Renaissance Medicine?"

12   The MNT Editorial Team, "What Is European Medieval and Renaissance Medicine?"

13   History.com Staff, "Black Death," A&E Television Networks, 2010, accessed July 1, 2017, http://www.history.com/topics/black-death.

14   The MNT Editorial Team, "What Is European Medieval & Renaissance Medicine?"

15   The MNT Editorial Team, "What Is European Medieval & Renaissance Medicine?"

Chapter 2

1   The MNT Editorial Team, "What Is Modern Medicine?" *Healthline Media*, last modified January 5, 2016, accessed July 1, 2017, http://www.medicalnewstoday.com/info/medicine/modern-medicine.php.

2   The MNT Editorial Team, "What Is Modern Medicine?"

3   The MNT Editorial Team, "What Is Modern Medicine?"

4   The MNT Editorial Team, "What Is Modern Medicine?"

5   Ed Smith, "Willow Meadowsweet Compound," *WordPress, Inc.*, last modified October 10, 2016, accessed July 7, 2017, http://www.herbaled.org/thm/compounds/will_meadow.html.

6   *Encyclopedia Britannica*, s.v. "Penicillin," last modified January 1, 2017, accessed July 29, 2017, https://www.britannica.com/science/penicillin#ref33693.

7   *Encyclopedia Britannica*, s.v. "Penicillin."

8   *New World Encyclopedia*, s.v. "Acetaminophen," last modified February 11, 2016, accessed July 29, 2017, http://www.newworldencyclopedia.org/entry/Acetaminophen.

9   Sandy McDowell, "What Is Methemoglobinemia?" *Healthline Media*, last modified June 19, 2017, accessed July 29, 2017, http://www.healthline.com/health/methemoglobinemia.

10   Jewish Virtual Library Staff, "Julius Axelrod," American-Israeli Cooperative Enterprise, accessed July 29, 2017, http://www.jewishvirtuallibrary.org/julius-axelrod.

11   *Encyclopedia.com*, s.v. "Tetracyclines," accessed October 30, 2017, http://www.encyclopedia.com/medicine/drugs/pharmacology/tetracycline.

12   "Lloyd Conover," Massachusetts Institute of Technology, accessed July 29, 2017, http://lemelson.mit.edu/resources/lloyd-conover.

13   The MNT Editorial Team, "What Is Modern Medicine?"

14   The MNT Editorial Team, "What Is Modern Medicine?"

15   History.com Staff, "The 1950s," A& E Networks, 2010, accessed June 29, 2017, http://www.history.com/topics/1950s#.

16   "The 1950s."

17   History.com Staff, "The 1960s," A& E Networks, 2010, accessed June 29, 2017, http://www.history.com/topics/1960s.

18   Allan Horwitz, "Book Review," *The New England Journal of Medicine*, February 19, 2009, accessed June 29, 2017, http://www.nejm.org/doi/pdf/10.1056/NEJMbkrev0809177.

19   Ivan Oransky, "Leo H. Steinbach," *The Lancets,* 366 (October 2005): 1430, http://www.thelancet.com/pdfs/journals/lancet/PIIS0140-6736(05)67588-5.pdf.

20   Claudia Campo-Soria, Yongchang Chang, and David S Weiss. "Mechanism of Action of Benzodiazepines on $GABA_A$ Receptors," *British Journal of Pharmacology* 148.7, (2006): 984–990, accessed October 31, 2017, https://www.ncbi.nlm.nih.gov/pmc/articles/PMC1751932/.

21   Laura Perez-Caballero et al., "Fluoxetine: A Case History of Its Discovery and Preclinical Development," *Expert Opinion on Drug Discovery* 9, no. 5 (2014): 567–578, https://doi.org/10.1517/17460441.2014.907790.

22   Francisco Lopez-Munoz and Cecilio Alamo, "Monoaminergic Neurotransmission: The History of the Discovery of Antidepressants from 1950s Until Today," *Current Pharmaceutical Design* 15, no. 14 (2009): 1563–1586, https://www.biopsychiatry.com/antidepressants.pdf.

23   The MNT Editorial Team, "What Is Modern Medicine?"

24   Akira Endo, "A Historical Perspective on the Discovery of Statins," *Japan Academy* 86, no. 5 (2010): 484–493, https://www.ncbi.nlm.nih.gov/pmc/articles/PMC3108295/pdf/pjab-86-484.pdf.

25   Endo, "A Historical Perspective on the Discovery of Statins," 484-493.

26   Endo, "A Historical Perspective on the Discovery of Statins," 484-493.
27   Endo, "A Historical Perspective on the Discovery of Statins," 484-493.
28   Ehrlich, "Herbal Medicine."

Chapter 3

1   LeafTV Contributor, "Where Does Pepper Come From?" *LeafTV*, 2007, accessed July 1, 2017, https://www.leaf.tv/articles/where-does-pepper-come-from/.

2   Bethany Moncel, "Classic Spice and Herb Blend," *TheSpruce*, last modified November 3, 2016, accessed July 1, 2017, https://www.thespruce.com/classic-spice-and-herb-blends-1328612.

3   Amanda Briney, "Geography of South Africa," *Thoughtco*, last modified March 3, 2017, accessed July 1, 2017, https://www.thoughtco.com/geography-of-south-africa-1435514?utm_term=history+south+africa&utm_content=p1-main-1title&utm_medium=sem&utm_source=gemini_s&utm_campaign=adid-04417bd1-47d6-4019-b597-39089f4be20f-0-ab_tsb_ocode-28735&ad=semD&an=gemini_s&am=broad&q=history+south+africa&o=28735&qsrc=999&l=sem&askid=04417bd1-47d6-4019-b597-39089f4be20f-0-ab_tsb.

4   History.com Staff, "The Gold Rush of 1849," A& E Networks, 2010, accessed July 1, 2017, http://www.history.com/topics/gold-rush-of-1849.

5   Chris Woodford, "Paint," *Explainthatstuff*, last modified December 9, 2016, accessed July 1, 2017, http://www.explainthatstuff.com/howpaintworks.html.

Chapter 4

1   "Heal." Merriam-Webster.com. Accessed November 1, 2017. https://www.merriam-webster.com/dictionary/heal.

2   "Minister." Merriam-Webster.com. Accessed November 1, 2017. https://www.merriam-webster.com/dictionary/minister.

Chapter 5

1   Merriam-Webster, "heal."
2   "What Is Cortisol?" *The Hormone Health Network*, accessed July 1, 2017, https://www.hormone.org/hormones-and-health/hormones/cortisol.
3   "Healthy Aging," *Johns Hopkins Medicine*, accessed July 1, 2017, http://www.hopkinsmedicine.org/health/healthy_aging/healthy_connections/forgiveness-your-health-depends-on-it.